THE ULTIMATE
KETOGENIC DIET

30 POUNDS IN 30 DAYS

JANE ARDANA

Table of Contents

Chapter 1: The Keto Plan & How it Works

You will soon understand how you can eat most of the foods you always enjoy. You will be able to make some substitutes to get going which are described within this chapter.

Happy Discovery!

Several Types of Keto Diet Plans

- *Plan 1*: You can choose from the standard ketogenic diet (SKD) which consists of high-fat, moderate protein, and is extremely low in carbs.

- *Plan 2*: The cyclical ketogenic diet or CKD is created with 5-keto days trailed by two high-carb days.

- *Plan 3*: The targeted keto diet, which is also called TKD, will provide you with a plan to add carbs to the diet during the times when you are working out.

- *Plan 4*: The high-protein ketogenic diet is very similar to the standard keto plan in all aspects except that it has more protein.

However, let's not get too far ahead of the plan. You need to focus on the first 30 days! The long process to explain each of these types would take another entire book!

Health Benefits from a Ketogenic Diet Plan

These are just a few of the ways you can benefit from remaining on the diet plan. It's hard to believe a diet plan can remedy so many health issues.

Acne: Your insulin levels are lowered by consuming less sugar and eating less processed foods. The acne will begin to clear up as you continue with the plan.

Alzheimer's disease: The symptoms and progression will be slowed.

Lowered Blood Pressure: While using the keto plan; you are experiencing reduced intake of carbs which will reduce your blood pressure levels. It is recommended to seek advice from your regular doctor to see if it is possible to reduce some of your medication while you are on the keto diet. You may also have some dizziness when you first begin the plan which is one of the first indications that the plan is working. The result is a lack of carbohydrates.

Cancer: Slow tumor growths and several other types of cancer have shown improvement with the keto plan.

Diabetes and Pre-diabetes: The main link to pre-diabetes is excess body fat which is removed which is proven by research that insulin sensitivity was improved by as much as 70%.

Epilepsy: Children's research studies have proven the diet works in the reduction of seizure activity.

Gum Disease: The sugar you consume influences the pH balance in your mouth. If you have issues before you begin the plan; you should begin to see a remarkable improvement within approximately three months.

Obesity: When the ketogenic diet plan is followed—the weight will dissolve.

Stiffness and Joint Pain: It is important to continue with the elimination of any grain-based foods. It is believed that the grains are one of the largest factors which cause the pain. Just remember "no grain—no pain."

Thinking is Improved: You might be a bit foggy-minded when you first begin the plan since you will be consuming high-fat foods. After all, your brain is about 60% fat by weight; your thinking skills should improve with the intake of the fatty foods indicated with the keto diet.

The Elements of Ketosis

Ketosis is used to help your burn body fat and drop extra pounds. Proteins will fuel your body to burn the fat—therefore—the ketosis will maintain your muscles and make you less hungry.

Your body will remain healthy and work as it should. If you don't consume enough carbs from your food; your cells will begin to burn fat for the necessary energy instead. Your body will switch over to ketosis for its energy source as your cut back on your calories and carbs.

Two elements that occur when your body doesn't need the glucose:

Lipogenesis: If there is a sufficient supply of glycogen in your liver and muscles, any excess is converted to fat and stored.

Glycogenesis: The excess of glucose converts to glycogen and is stored in the muscles and liver. Research indicates that only about half of your energy used daily can be stored as glycogen.

As a result, your body will have no more food—similar to when you are sleeping—your body burns the fat and creates ketones. These ketones break down the fats, which generate fatty acids, and burn-off in the liver through beta-oxidation.

Simply stated, when you no longer have a supply of glycogen or glucose, ketosis begins and will use the consumed/stored fat as energy.

The Internet provides you with a keto calculator to use at http://keto-calculator.ankerl.com/. You can check your levels when you want to know what essentials your body needs during your diet plan or after. All you need to do is document your personal information such as weight and height. The calculator will provide you with the essential math.

Weight Loss and Protein

Protein needs to be in your plan for these reasons:

Protein is a Fat Burner: Science has proven your body cannot use and burn your fat as energy sources unless you have help from either carbs or protein. The balance of protein must be maintained to preserve your calorie-burning lean muscles.

Protein Saves Your Calories: Protein slows down your digestion process making you feel more satisfied from the foods you eat. During the first cycle of your diet plan; it is imperative that you feel full, so there is no temptation to cheat on the strategy.

Muscle Repair and Growth: Protein should be increased on days when you are more active. It is essential to have a plan on what your meals will consist of with a balance of carbs, proteins, and calories. The balance is what you are attempting to achieve with a focused plan such as the keto diet.

The Role of Calories, Protein, and Carbs

Calories are held within your body with the use of the nutrients of protein, fat, and carbs which your body will use for energy.

Carbohydrates

Your body exchanges one-hundred percent of the carbs into glucose which gives your body an energy boost. About 50% to 60% of your intake of calories is produced by carbs. Carbs stored in your liver as glycogen is released as your body needs it. Glucose is essential for the creation of adenosine triphosphate (ATP) which is an energy molecule. The fuel from glucose is vital for the daily maintenance and activities inside your body. After the liver has reached its maximum capacity for its limits, the excessive carbohydrates turn into fat.

Count Those Carbs

Before you are totally in gear, you need to start carb counting to make sure you keep your body in perfect 'sync' with the plan. Reading the labels may be a bit nerve-racking in the beginning, but after a while, it will be as you have always done it that way.

Remember this Formula: Total Carbs minus (-) Fiber = Net Carbs

A rough estimate will include you consuming between 20 to 30 carbs daily. It is almost a necessity to own a set of food scales to take out the guesswork.

Keep this information in mind before you make the purchase:

- *The Automatic Shut-Off*: Seek a scale that does not have this option. The result could be you being in the midst of a recipe—move the dish—and the scale could reset; NOT.

- *The Tare Function*: When you set a bowl on the scale, the feature will allow you to reset the scale back to zero (0).

- *Removable Plate*: Keep the germs off of the scale by removing the plate. Be sure it will come off to eliminate the bacterial buildup.

- *Seek a Conversion Button*: You need to know how to convert measurements into grams since not all recipes have them listed. The grams keep the system in complete harmony.

Natural Supplements for Ketogenic Dieters

Fermented Foods: Use items, while on the keto plan such as coconut milk kefir, coconut milk, yogurt, pickles, sauerkraut, and kimchi to help with any digestive issues.

Lemon and Lime: Your blood sugar levels will naturally drop with these citric additions, and signal a boost in your liver function. Use them in green juices, with a salad, or with cooked with meats or veggies. The choices are limitless and assist you with the following:

- Reduces toothache pain

- Boosts your immune system

- Relieves respiratory infections

- Balances pH

- Decreases wrinkles and blemishes

- Reduces fever

- Excellent for weight loss

- Flushes out the unwanted, unhealthy materials

- Blood purifier

Apple Cider Vinegar: Who would believe the benefits you can receive from just one to two tablespoons of vinegar in an 8-ounce glass of water would help the process? You can choose the straight up method and skip the water. These are just a few ways this helps your progress:

- Reduces cholesterol

- Excellent for detoxification

- Helps you to drop the pounds

- Improves your digestion tract

- Helps with sore muscles

- Controls sugar intake/aids in diabetes

- Strengthens your immune system

- A good energy booster

- Balances your inner body system and functions

Cinnamon: Use cinnamon as part of your daily plan to improve your insulin receptor activity. Just put one-half of a teaspoon of cinnamon into a shake or any type of keto dessert. Many of the keto recipes contain the ingredient.

Turmeric: Dating back to Ayurveda and Chinese medicine the is of this Asian orange herb has been known for its anti-inflammatory compounds.

Add it to you smoothies, green drinks, meats, or veggies. These are some of its benefits:

- Prevents Alzheimer's disease

- Weight management

- Relieves arthritis

- Reduces your cholesterol levels

- Helps control diabetes

- Improves your digestion

Be Aware of Some Foods and Beverages: Which Ones to Avoid

Agave Nectar: One teaspoon has 5 grams of carbs versus 4 grams in table sugar.

Beans and Legumes: This group to avoid includes peas, lentils, kidney beans, and chickpeas. If you use them, be sure to count the carbs, protein, and fat content.

Cashews and Pistachios: The high carb content should be monitored for these yummy nuts.

Fruits: Raspberries, blueberries, and cranberries contain high sugar contents. In small portions; you can enjoy some strawberries.

Grains and Starches: Avoid wheat-based items such as cereal, rice, or pasta.

Hydrogenated Fats: Cold-pressed items should be avoided when using vegetable oils such as safflower, olive, soybean, or flax. Coronary heart disease has been linked to these fats which also include margarine.

Tomato-based Products: Read the labels because most of the tomato products contain sugar. If you use them be sure to account for the sugar content. (The recipes provided have considered this.)

Chapter 2: The 14-Day Plan

Day One

Breakfast: Keto Scrambled Eggs

Ingredients

3 large eggs

Fresh ground pepper

Coarse salt

1 tablespoon unsalted butter

Instructions

1. Whisk the eggs in a bowl.

2. Use low heat and place the butter into a skillet.

3. Add the eggs. Continue to stir until well-done, usually 1 ½ to 3 minutes.

Serving Portion: Fat: 26.3 g; Carbs 1.8 g; Protein: 17.4 g; Calories: 318

Lunch: Tuna Cheese Melt (Low-Carbs)

Ingredients

2 Pieces of "Oopsie" bread

Ingredients for the Salad

1 to 2 Celery stalks

5 1/3 Tablespoons sour cream or mayonnaise

1 Can tuna (in olive oil)

4 Tablespoons chopped dill pickles

½ teaspoon lemon juice

Pepper and salt to taste

½ minced clove garlic

Toppings

A pinch of paprika powder or cayenne pepper

3 ½ ounces shredded cheese

Serving Ingredients

Olive oil

1/3 Pound leafy greens

"Oopsie" Bread (makes six to 8)

3 Eggs

A pinch of salt

4 ¼ ounces cream cheese

½ teaspoon baking powder

½ Tablespoon ground psyllium husk powder

Instructions

1. Preheat the oven to 350°F. Put parchment paper onto a cookie sheet.

2. Blend all of the salad ingredients.

3. Place the bread slices on the prepared sheet, spread the tuna, and sprinkle the cheese on top of each slice of bread.

4. Sprinkle some cayenne or paprika powder on the sandwich halves and bake in the oven for about 15 minutes.

5. Have some leafy greens with a drizzle of olive oil.

"Oopsie" Bread Instructions

1. Heat the oven to oven at 300°F.

2. Begin by separating the egg whites (whites in one bowl and yolks in the other).

3. Whisk the egg whites with the salt until peaks are formed.

4. Combine the cream cheese and egg yolks—add the baking powder and psyllium seed husk (making it more Oopsie type bread).

5. Blend/fold in the whites into the yolk mixture—keeping out the air in the whites of the eggs.

6. Place six or eight 'oopsies' on the paper-lined sheet.

7. Bake in the center oven rack, usually for 25 minutes or until browned.

Dinner: Chicken Smothered in Creamy Onion Sauce

Ingredients

1 whole green/spring onion

2 tablespoons or 1-ounce butter

4 chicken breast halves (skinless—boneless)

8 ounces sour cream

½ teaspoon sea salt

Note: The chicken should weigh approximately six ounces or 170 g for this recipe.

Instructions

1. In a large pan, melt the butter on the stovetop using the med-high setting. Lower the heat setting to med-low—put the chicken with the butter—cover and cook about ten more minutes.

2. Chop the onion using just the white and green sections.

3. Flip the breasts—cover and simmer—another 8 or 9 minutes (or until completely done).

4. Combine the onion, and continue cooking the chicken for another one or two minutes.

5. Take it off of the burner, and blend in the salt and sour cream.

6. Let the meal rest and flavors blend for five minutes.

Stir well and serve.

Day Two

Breakfast: Mock Mc Griddle Casserole

Ingredients

1 pound breakfast sausage

¼ cup flaxseed meal

1 cup almond flour

10 large eggs

6 tablespoons maple syrup

4 ounces cheese

4 tablespoons butter

¼ teaspoon sage

½ teaspoon each: onion & garlic powder

Instructions

1. Heat the oven to 350°F. Use parchment paper to line a 9 x 9-inch casserole dish.

2. Using medium heat; start cooking the breakfast sausage on the stove in a skillet.

3. Blend all of the dry (the cheese included) ingredients and add the wet ones.

4. Add four tablespoons of the syrup and blend well.

5. After the sausage is crispy brown—blend all of the ingredients; (the fat too).

6. Pour the mixture into the dish and sprinkle the remainder of the syrup on the top.

7. Bake for 45 to 55 minutes. Remove it and let it cool.

Yields: Eight Servings

Time Saving Tip: The casserole should be easy to remove by using the edge of the parchment paper.

Lunch: Brussels Sprouts with Hamburger Gratin

Ingredients

1 Pound Ground beef

1 Pound Brussels sprouts

½ Pound diced bacon

4 tablespoons sour cream

1/3 Pound shredded cheese

1- ¾ Ounces butter

Pepper and salt to taste

1 tablespoon Italian seasoning

Instructions

1. Cut the Brussels sprouts in half.
2. Preheat the oven to 425°F/220°C.
3. Saute the Brussels sprouts and bacon in the butter. Flavor with the sour cream and place in a baking pan/dish.
4. Fry the beef and season with pepper and salt; add the herbs and cheese—sprinkling on top of the base layer.
5. Bake on the center rack of the oven for fifteen minutes.

Serve with a dollop of mayonnaise and a fresh salad.

Yields: Four Servings

Dinner: Squash and Sausage Casserole

Ingredients

1 pound browned sausage

2 large eggs

1 medium zucchini (sliced & cooked)

2 medium summer squash (sliced & cooked)

1 teaspoon salt

½ teaspoon onion powder or ¼ cup dried minced onion

1 cup mayonnaise

1 package sugar substitute (or stevia)

¼ teaspoon pepper

1 ½ cups shredded cheddar cheese (divided)

¼ melted butter

Instructions

1. Pre-set the oven to 350°F.

2. Blend each of the ingredients except for one-half of a cup of shredded cheese.

3. Put the ingredients into a lightly greased oblong baking plate.

4. Sprinkle the remainder of cheese on the casserole.

5. Bake until lightly browned for approximately thirty minutes.

This casserole will easily serve 12 people with an amazing flavor you won't soon forget!

Day Three

Breakfast: Can't Beat it Porridge

Ingredients

1 cups almond or coconut milk

1 pinch salt

1 Tablespoon each:

- Sunflower seeds
- Chia Seeds

Instructions

1. Using a small saucepan on the stovetop, blend each of the components, and bring to a boiling. Lower the burner and cook slowly until the porridge is the consistency you desire

2. Garnish with some butter or milk. You can also add some fresh unsweetened berries or cinnamon.

Yields: One Serving

Time Saving Tip: Make it ahead of time using a big glass jar. Fill the jar with the following ingredients and shake them up. Each serving will correspond with three tablespoons for each serving.

These are the ingredients needed for the batch:

1 Tbsp. cinnamon

½ tsp. salt

1 1/4 cup each:

- Sunflower seeds

- Flaxseeds

- Chia seeds

Lunch: Salad From a Jar

Ingredients

1 (4-ounce) rotisserie chicken/smoked salmon/other protein

1 ounce each:

- Cucumber

- Cherry tomatoes

- Leafy greens

- Bell pepper

4 tablespoons olive oil or mayonnaise

½ Scallion

Instructions

1. Chop or shred the veggies and place the leafy greens to the bottom for a crunch followed by the colorful veggies. (You can also use some cauliflower or broccoli for a change of pace.)

2. Top it off with some of the grilled protein of your choice. You can also use cold cuts, tuna fish, mackerel or boiled eggs.

3. Cheese cubes, seeds, nuts, and olives are also healthy and colorful additions.

4. Add a generous amount of mayonnaise or salad dressing and enjoy!

Yields: One Serving

Dinner: Ham and Cheese Stromboli

Ingredients

1 large egg

1 ¼ cups shredded mozzarella cheese

3 tablespoons coconut flour

4 tablespoons almond flour

4 ounces of ham

1 teaspoon Italian seasoning

3 ½ ounces cheddar cheese

Instructions

1. Preheat the oven to 400°F.

2. Melt the mozzarella cheese in the microwave for one minute/alternating at ten-second intervals; stirring until melted.

3. In a mixing bowl, blend the coconut and almond flour with the seasonings.

4. Toss in the mozzarella on the top and work it in.

5. After the cheese has cooled; beat the egg and combine everything

6. On a flat surface; put some parchment paper, and add the mixture.

7. Use a rolling pin or your hands to flatten the mix.

8. Place several diagonal lines using a knife or pizza cutter. (Leave a row of approximately four inches wide in the center.

9. Alternate the layers using the cheddar and ham on the uncut space of dough until you have used all of the filling.

10. Bake for 15 to 20minutes or it is browned.

Day Four

Breakfast: Frittata with Cheese and Tomatoes

Ingredients

6 eggs

2/3 cup soft cheese (ex. Feta 3 ½ ounces or 100 g)

½ medium white onion (1.9 ounces or 55 g)

2/3 cup halved cherry tomatoes

2 tablespoons chopped herbs (ex. basil or chives)

1 tablespoon ghee/butter

Instructions

1. Heat the oven broiler to 400°F.

2. Place the onions on a greased, hot iron skillet, and cook with ghee/butter until slightly brown.

3. In a separate container, crack the eggs and add the salt, pepper, or add herbs of your choice. Whisk and add to the onion pan.

4. Cook until the edges begin to get brown. Top with the cheese and tomatoes.

5. Put the pan in the broiler for five to seven minutes or until done.

Lunch: Chicken—Broccoli—Zucchini Boats

For a variety textures as well as flavors to spice up lunch; this is the one!

Ingredients

6 ounces shredded chicken

2 tablespoons butter

2 hollowed-out zucchini (10 ounces)

3 ounces shredded cheddar cheese

1 stalk of green onion

1 cup broccoli

2 tablespoons sour cream

Instructions

1. Heat the oven temperature to 400°F.

2. Slice the zucchini lengthwise and scoop most of the insides out until you have a shell of approximately ½ to 1 cm. thick.

3. Melt one tablespoon of the butter into each boat, flavor with a dash of pepper and salt, and bake them for around twenty minutes.

4. Shred the chicken, cut the broccoli florets into small pieces, and measure out six ounces of cheese. Blend in with the sour cream.

5. Remove the zucchini shells when done and add the mixture.

6. Sprinkle each of them with the remainder of the cheese.

7. Bake for another ten or fifteen minutes until the cheese is browned and melted.

8. Use a bit of sour cream, mayonnaise, or chopped onion as a garnish.

Dinner: Steak-Lovers Slow-Cooked Chili

Ingredients for Chili:

1 cup beef or chicken stock

½ cup sliced leeks

2 ½ pounds (1-inch cubes) steak

2 cups whole tomatoes (canned with juices)

1 tablespoon chili powder

½ tsp. salt

1/8 tsp. ground black pepper

¼ tsp. ground cayenne pepper

½ tsp. cumin

Optional Toppings

1 teaspoon fresh chopped cilantro

2 tablespoons sour cream

¼ cup shredded cheddar cheese

½ avocado (cubed or sliced)

Instructions

1. Place all of the items except the topping fixings into the slow cooker.

2. Set the cooker on the high setting for about six hours.

Yields: Twelve Servings

Serving Portion: 1: Fat: 26.0 g; Carbs 3.3 g; Protein: 38.4 g; Calories: 321

Servings with Toppings: Serving Portion: 1: Fat: 41.32 g; Carbs 13.49 g; Protein: 32.47 g; Calories: 540.33

Day 5

Breakfast: Brownie Muffins

Ingredients

½ tsp. salt

1 cup flaxseed meal

¼ cup cocoa powder

½ Tbsp. baking powder

1 Tbsp. cinnamon

2 Tbsp. coconut oil

1 large egg

1 tsp. vanilla extract

¼ cup sugar-free caramel syrup

½ cup pumpkin puree

¼ cup slivered almonds

1 tsp. apple cider vinegar

Instructions

1. Heat the oven temperature at 350°F.

2. In a deep mixing bowl—combine all of the ingredients—mixing well.

3. Use six paper liners in the muffin tin, and add ¼ cup of the batter to each one.

4. Sprinkle several almonds on the tops, pressing gently.

5. Bake approximately fifteen minutes. It is done when the top is set.

Serving Portion: 1 muffin (The recipe serves six): Fat: 13.4 g; Carbs 8.2 g; Protein: 7 g; Calories: 183.3

Lunch: Bacon-Avocado-Goat Cheese Salad

Ingredients

½ Pound bacon

½ Pound goat cheese

4 ounces walnuts

2 avocados

4 ounces arugula lettuce

Ingredients for the Dressing

7 ½ tablespoons mayonnaise

Juice of ½ of a lemon

2 tablespoons heavy whipping cream

7 ½ tablespoons olive oil

Instructions

1. Preheat the oven temperature to 400°F/200°C.

2. Prepare a baking dish with some parchment paper.

3. Slice the goat cheese into ½-inch round slices and put in the baking dish. Place on the upper rack of the oven.

4. Pan-fry the bacon until crunchy.

5. Cut the avocados and place on top of a bed of lettuce, add the bacon, cheese, and nuts to the top of your creation.

6. Make the dressing using a stick blender. Sprinkle in a dash of pepper, salt, or a few fresh herbs.

Yields: Four Servings

Dinner: Tenderloin Stuffed Keto Style

Ingredients

2 pounds pork tenderloin or venison

½ cup feta cheese

½ cup gorgonzola cheese

1 teaspoon chopped onion

2 tablespoons crushed almonds

2 garlic cloves, minced

½ teaspoon each: fresh ground black pepper and sea salt

Instructions

1. Preheat the grill.

2. Form a pocket in the tenderloin.

3. Mix the cheeses, almonds, garlic, and onions.

4. Stuff the pocket, and seal using a skewer.

5. Grill until its desired doneness.

Yields: Eight Servings

Serving Portion: 1: Fat: 6.2 g; Carbs 2.9 g; Protein: 28.8 g; Calories: 194

Day 6

Breakfast: Sausage—Feta—Spinach Omelet

Ingredients

½ tablespoon extra-virgin olive oil

2 sausage links

3 large eggs

¼ cup Half & Half

1 cup spinach

1 tablespoon feta cheese

Note: You will need two skillets for this yummy omelet!

Instructions

1. Use medium heat for both pans, and pour olive oil in one of the two.

2. In a small dish, use the Half & Half and mix with the eggs—add the seasonings—and scramble.

3. In the clean pan, cook the sausage.

4. Sauté the spinach in the oiled pan—add a pinch of salt and pepper if desired.

5. After both have finished cooking; put them together in a bowl.

6. Transfer the olive oiled pan to the sausage fat pan—and add the eggs.

7. When the edges begin to cook—add the spinach, sausage, and cheese. Cook another minute—flip the omelet. Cook another two to three minutes.

8.   Cover one pan with the other and let the combo steam.

9.   Remove and enjoy your masterpiece!

Serving Portion: Fat: 43 g; Carbs 3 g; Protein: 31 g; Calories: 535

Lunch: Pancakes with Cream-Cheese Topping

Don't be alarmed, this is an excellent choice for any time and is so healthy.

Ingredients

8 ¾ ounces cottage cheese

5 eggs

1 tablespoon ground psyllium husk powder

A pinch of salt

For Frying: Coconut oil or butter

Ingredients for the Topping

2 tablespoons red or green pesto

½ pound (8 ounces) ricotta or cream cheese

2 tablespoons olive oil

Ground black pepper and Sea Salt

½ thinly sliced red onion

Instructions

1.   Combine one tablespoon of the olive oil with the pesto and cream cheese; set aside.

2.   Using a hand blender, mix the salt, cottage cheese, eggs, and husk powder; blend until smooth. Let rest for ten minutes.

3.   On the stovetop using the medium heat setting; heat two tablespoons of the oil or butter.

4. Drop several dollops of the cheese batter (2 to 3 inches in diameter), frying the pancakes a few minutes per side.

5. Serve with a few red onion slices with a drizzle of oil, pepper, and salt. You can also use fresh herbs, smoked fish roe or chopped chives.

Dinner: Skillet Style Sausage and Cabbage Melt

Ingredients

4 spicy Italian chicken sausages

2 tablespoons coconut oil

½ cup diced onion

1 ½ cups purple cabbage

1 ½ cups green cabbage

2 tablespoons chopped fresh cilantro

2-1-ounce slices Colby jack cheese

Instructions

1. Start by removing the sausage casings and rough-chopping them. Shred the cabbage and chop the onions.

2. Add the coconut oil, cabbage, and onion in a large skillet using the med-high setting for approximately eight minutes (the veggies should be tender).

3. Blend the cheese and cover.

4. Turn the heat off and let it rest five minutes as the cheese melts.

5. When it is time to serve—stir gently and add the cilantro.

Yields: Four Servings

Serving Portion: 1: Fat: 14.62 g; Carbs 3.52 g; Protein: 18.26 g; Calories: 231

Day 7

Breakfast: Tapas

Have a great mixture!

Ingredients

Cold Cuts:

- Prosciutto
- Serrano ham
- Salami
- Chorizo

Cheeses:

- Gouda
- Parmesan
- Mozzarella
- Cheddar

Veggies:

- Pickled cucumbers
- Peppers
- Radishes
- Cucumbers

Avocado with pepper and homemade mayonnaise

Fresh Basil

Splash of fresh squeezed lemon juice

Nuts:

- Hazelnuts

- Almonds

- Walnuts

Instructions

1. Cut all of the ingredients into cubes or sticks and split the avocado cutting its fruit into small wedges.

2. Blend with four ounces of mayonnaise pepper and maybe a splash of lemon juice

3. Use the avocado shells for the serving platter.

Yields: Four Servings

Lunch: Tofu—Bok-Choy Salad

Tofu Ingredients:

15 ounces extra firm tofu

2 teaspoons minced garlic

Juice from ½ a lemon

1 tablespoon each:

- sesame oil

- water

- soy sauce

- rice wine vinegar

Bok Choy Salad Ingredients:

2 tablespoons soy sauce

1 stalk green onion

2 tablespoons chopped cilantro

9 ounces bok choy

3 tablespoons coconut oil

1 tablespoon Sambal Olek

Juice of ½ of a lime

1 tablespoon peanut butter

7 drops liquid Stevia

Instructions

1. Press the tofu in towels for approximately five to six hours to dry.

2. Combine each of the marinade ingredients.

3. When dry; chop the tofu into squares and put in a plastic container/bag with the marinade sauce.

4. Leave it to sit for at least thirty minutes—preferably overnight.

5. Heat the oven to 350°F. Bake for 30 to 35 minutes on a parchment paper-lined baking dish or a Silpat (non-stick baking sheet with a blend of fiberglass mesh and silicone).

6. In the interim, combine the dressing ingredients (except for the bok choy) in a mixing dish. Toss in the onion and cilantro.

7. Chop the bok choy as you would cabbage, into small slices.

8. Remove the tofu—combine, and enjoy.

Note: Bok choy is a Chinese vegetable.

Serving Portion: Fat: 35 g; Carbs 7.3 g; Protein: 25.0 g; Calories: 442.3

Dinner: Hamburger Stroganoff

Ingredients

8 ounces sliced mushrooms

1 pound ground beef

2 minced cloves of garlic

2 Tbsp. butter

1 ¼ cups sour cream

1/3 cup water or dry white wine

1 tsp. lemon juice

¼ tsp. paprika

1 tsp. dried parsley

Substitute: You may also use one tablespoon fresh chopped parsley.

Instructions

1. Sauté the onions and garlic in a skillet prepared using one tablespoon of butter.

2. Mix in the beef into the pan— sprinkle with pepper and salt if desired. Cook until done and set to the side.

3. Use the remainder of the butter, the mushrooms, and the wine/water, and add them to the pan. Cook until half of the liquid is reduced and the mushrooms are soft.

4. Take them off the burner—add the paprika and sour cream.

5. On low heat stir in the meat and lemon juice.

Use additional spices for flavoring if desired.

Serving Portion: 1 (272 g): Fat: 28.1 g; Carbs 6.1 g; Protein: 38.7 g; Calories: 447

Day 8

Breakfast: Cheddar—Jalapeno Waffles

Ingredients

3 large eggs

1 small jalapeno

3 ounces cream cheese

1 tablespoon coconut flour

1-ounce cheddar cheese

1 teaspoon each:

- baking powder
- Psyllium husk powder

Instructions

1. Combine all of the ingredients using an immersion blender (except for the jalapeno and cheese) until it has a smooth texture.

2. Add the cheese and jalapeno; blend and pour into the waffle iron.

3. You can garnish with your favorite ingredients in about five or six minutes total

Note: Psyllium husk is a native of Pakistan, Bangladesh, and India. It is available online at several locations

Serving Portion: 2 waffles: Fat: 28 g; Carbs 6 g; Protein: 16 g; Calories: 338

Lunch: Salmon Tandoori with Cucumber Sauce

Ingredients

1 ½ Pounds Salmon (In pieces)

2 tablespoons coconut oil

1 tablespoon tandoori seasoning

Ingredients for the Cucumber Sauce

½ cup shredded cucumber

1 ¼ cup sour cream or mayonnaise

2 minced garlic cloves

Juice of ½ of a lime

Optional: ½ teaspoon salt

Ingredients for the Crispy Salad

3 ½ ounces arugula lettuce

3 scallions

1 yellow pepper

Juice of 1 lime

2 avocados

Instructions

1. Preheat the oven to 350°F.

2. Mix the tandoori seasoning and the 2 tablespoons of oil to coat the salmon.

3. Bake the salmon for fifteen to twenty minutes.

4. Combine the lime juice, garlic, cucumber (blot the water out with paper towels first), and sour cream/mayonnaise in a mixing dish.

5. Prepare the salad ingredients and enjoy.

Yields: Four Servings

Dinner: Ground Beef Stir Fry

Ingredients

300 g (approximately 10 ½ ounces) ground beef

5 medium brown mushrooms

½ cup broccoli

2 leaves kale

½ medium Spanish onion

1 Tbsp. coconut oil

½ medium red pepper

1 Tbsp. cayenne pepper

1 Tbsp. Chinese Five Spices

Note: McCormick was used for the Five Spices

Instructions

1. Prepare the vegetables—slice the mushrooms—chop the broccoli.

2. Heat a frying pan on the stovetop using the med-high setting. Pour in the oil and toss in the onions. Cook for an additional minute.

3. Blend the remainder of the vegetables and cook an additional two minutes—stirring often.

4. Combine the spices and beef—lower the heat to medium—and continue cooking for approximately two more minutes.

5. Cover the pan and cook for five or ten more minutes until the beef is done.

Serving Portion: 1 (Recipe is for three servings): Fat: 18 g; Carbs 7 g; Protein: 29 g; Calories: 307

Day 9

Breakfast: Cheddar and Sage Waffles

Ingredients

1 1/3 coconut flour

1 teaspoon ground sage

½ teaspoon salt

¼ teaspoon garlic powder

3 teaspoons baking powder

2 cups canned coconut milk

½ cup water

3 tablespoons melted coconut oil

1 cup shredded cheddar cheese

2 eggs

Instructions

1. Prepare the waffle iron on the required manufacturer's setting. Grease the iron (top and bottom).

2. Blend all of the seasonings, flour, and baking powder in a container.

3. Mix the wet ingredients, stirring until the batter becomes stiff. Blend in the cheese.

4. Scoop out a one-third cup of the batter and place in each section of the iron.

5. Depending on how you like your waffles; you can run them through two cycles on the iron if you want it crispier.

Serving Portion: 1 waffles (The recipe serves 12): Fat: 17.21 g; Carbs 9.2 g; Protein: 6.52 g; Calories: 213.97

Lunch: Crispy Shrimp Salad on an Egg Wrap

Ingredients for the Wraps

1-ounce butter

4 eggs

Pepper and salt to taste

Shrimp Salad Ingredients

6 ounces shrimp

2 avocados

1/2 of an apple/handful of radishes

1 teaspoon lime juice

1 celery stalk

1 cup mayonnaise

1 red chili pepper

8 tablespoons fresh parsley or cilantro

Instructions for the Wrap

1. Cook and peel the shrimp. Finely chop the red chili pepper and fresh cilantro/parsley.

2. Whip the eggs with the pepper and salt.

3. Using a medium frying pan, melt the butter. Empty half of the egg batter until the egg gets firm, and repeat for the second one.

Instructions for the Salad

1. Slice the avocado and scoop out providing you with ½-inch cubes. Place them in a dish and give a fresh squeeze of juice over them and mix.

2. Dice the apple and thinly slice the celery, putting them with the avocado. Blend in the peppers, cilantro/parsley, and mayonnaise.

3. Combine well and gently stir in the shrimps. Add more salt if desired.

Yields: Two Servings

This is one of those meals that can be enjoyed with leafy greens or alone. Add a couple of boiled eggs in place of the wrap for another healthy choice.

Dinner: Bacon Wrapped Meatloaf

Ingredients

1 finely chopped yellow onion

1 ½ Pounds ground lamb, poultry, pork *or* beef

2 tablespoons butter

8 tablespoons heavy whipping cream

1 egg

6 ¾ tablespoons shredded cheese

1 tablespoon dried basil/oregano

1 tsp. salt

½ tsp. black pepper

7 ¾ ounces sliced bacon

Optional: ½ tablespoon tamari soy sauce

For the Gravy: 1 ¼ cups heavy whipping cream

Instructions

1. Preheat the oven to 400°F/200°C.

2. Saute the onion in a pan with the butter, but don't brown it.

3. Combine the meat in a container, adding all of the remainders of ingredients but omit the bacon. Don't over-work it, but blend the ingredients well, making a loaf.

4. Bake it in the center of the oven for approximately 45 minutes. You can use some aluminum foil to cover the meatloaf, just in case, the bacon begins to scorch.

5. Reserve any of the accumulated juices and make the gravy, blending it with the cream in a small saucepan.

6. Let the mixture come to a boil using low heat until it is creamy and the right texture, usually for approximately ten to fifteen minutes.

7. Spice it up with a drizzle of tamari soy sauce for a bit of flavor.

8. Have some cauliflower or broccoli on the side with some butter. It is all up to you to decide on the veggie choices.

Yields: Four Servings

Day 10

Breakfast: Omelet Wrap with Avocado & Salmon

Ingredients

3 large eggs

½ package smoked salmon (100 g or 1.8 ounces)

½ avocado (3.5 ounces or 100 g)

1 spring onion (1/2 ounce or 15 g)

2 tablespoons cream cheese (full-fat—2.3 ounces or 64 g)

2 tablespoons chives (freshly chopped)

1 tablespoon butter or ghee

Instructions

1. In a mixing bowl—add a pinch of pepper and salt along with the eggs. Use a fork or whisk—mixing them well. Blend the chives and cream cheese.

2. Prepare the salmon and avocado (peel and slice).

3. In a sauté pan, melt the butter/ghee, and add the egg mixture. Cook until fluffy.

4. Put the omelet on a serving dish, and spoon the mixture of cheese over it.

5. Sprinkle the onion, prepared avocado, and salmon into the wrap.

Close and enjoy!

Serving Portion: Fat: 66.9g; Carbs 13.3 g; Protein: 36.9 g

Lunch: Tuna Avocado Melt

Ingredients

1-10 - ounce can drained tuna

1 medium cubed avocado

¼ cup mayonnaise

1/3 cup almond flour

¼ teaspoon onion powder

¼ cup parmesan cheese

½ teaspoon garlic powder

1/2 cup coconut oil (for frying)

Instructions

1. In a mixing container, blend all of the ingredients except for the coconut oil and avocado. Fold the cubed avocado into the tuna.

2. Make balls and coat each one with the almond flour.

3. Use the medium heat setting and put the oil in a pan—mix the tuna—and continue cooking until brown.

Note: Some people like to use this as a casserole dish.

Yields: Twelve Servings

Per Serving Portion: Fat: 11.8 g; Carbs 2.0 g; Protein: 6.2 g; Calories: 134.7

Dinner: Hamburger Patties with Fried Cabbage

Ingredients for the Hamburger Patties

1 egg

1 ½ Pounds ground beef

3 ¼ ounces feta cheese

1 tsp. salt

¼ tsp. ground black pepper

1 ¾ ounces finely- chopped, fresh parsley

1-ounce butter

1 tablespoon olive oil

Ingredients for the Gravy

1 ¾ - Ounces fresh (coarsely chopped) parsley

1 ¼ cups heavy whipping cream

Pepper and Salt

2 tablespoons tomato paste

Ingredients for the Green Cabbage

4 ¼ ounces butter

1 ½ Pounds shredded green cabbage

Pepper and Salt

Instructions

1. Form eight oblong patties by blending all of the ingredients listed under the hamburger patties.

2. Using the med-high setting on the stovetop, prepare a skillet with olive oil and butter and fry the patties for a minimum of ten minutes.

3. Empty the whipping cream and tomato paste into the mixture—stir—and let them blend.

Serve with some parsley for garnishment.

Instructions for Butter-fried Green Cabbage

1. Use a food processor or knife to shred the cabbage.

2. Prepare a frying pan with the butter and sauté the cabbage for approximately fifteen minutes on the med-high setting.

3. Reduce the heat for the last five minutes (or so)—stirring regularly.

Variations: You can also enjoy this with whatever you desire, including spinach, carrots, mushrooms, acorn squash, or corn.

Yields: Four Servings

Day 11

Breakfast: The Breadless Breakfast Sandwich

Ingredients

4 Eggs

1-ounce ham/pastrami cold cuts

2 tablespoons butter

2 ounces of edam/provolone/cheddar cheese

Several drops of Worcestershire or Tabasco sauce

Pepper and salt to taste

Instructions

1. Cut the cheese into thick slices.

2. Prepare a frying pan over medium heat. Fry the eggs over-easy with a pinch of pepper and salt.

3. Add the choice of meat onto the two eggs, a layer of cheese, and the egg for the top of the 'bun.'

4. Give the sandwich a splash of Worcestershire sauce/Tabasco and serve. You can also use some French Dijon mustard to complement the ham.

Yields: Two Servings

Lunch: Thai Fish With Coconut & Curry

Ingredients

1 ½ Pounds whitefish/salmon

4 tablespoons butter/ghee

Pepper and salt

1 to 2 tablespoons green/red curry paste

8 tablespoons fresh chopped cilantro

1 can coconut cream

1 Pound broccoli/cauliflower

For Greasing the Dish: Olive oil/butter

Instructions

1. Grease a baking dish. Preheat the oven to 400°F.

2. Place the salmon/fish in a dish where there is not any extra space between the dish and fish (not meant as a rhyme).

3. Place a dab of butter on each piece along with a shake of pepper and salt.

4. Combine the chopped cilantro, curry paste and coconut cream in a small container. Pour it over the fish.

5. Bake until the fish is falling apart done, usually about twenty minutes.

6. Boil the broccoli/cauliflower in water (lightly salted) for several minutes as a side dish.

Yields: Four Servings

Dinner: Keto Tacos or Nachos

Ingredients

500 g or 17.6 ounces ground beef

1 medium white onion (3.0 ounces)

4 tacos

1 teaspoon chili powder

2 garlic cloves

½ teaspoon ground cumin

2 teaspoons extra-virgin coconut oil or ghee

1 tablespoon unsweetened tomato puree

1 cup water (8 ounces)

½ teaspoon salt—more or less

Cayenne pepper or freshly ground black pepper

Topping Ingredients

1 small head of lettuce (approximately 3.5 ounces or 100 g)

1 cup or 5.3 ounces cherry tomatoes

1 medium avocado (7.1 ounces or 200 g)

Optional Toppings

4 tablespoons sour cream

1 cup grated cheese

Veggies including cabbage, cucumbers, or peppers

Instructions

1. Using med-high, add some butter/ghee in a frying pan; toss in the onion. Sauté until brown and mix in the beef, continue cooking until the beef is done.

2. Add the cumin and chili powder. (You can substitute with 1 ½ teaspoon of paprika.)

3. Pour in the water and add the tomato puree. Also add pepper, and salt if you like for additional flavoring.

4. Continue cooking until the meat is done and approximately ¼ of the sauce is reduced. Set to the side and prepare the vegetable topping.

5. Use the meat mixture to stuff the shells. Garnish with some of the tomatoes, lettuce, and avocado.

6. As an option, you can add a bit of sour cream or cheddar cheese.

Note: You may use this as a tasty taco or on the side with the meat as the centerfold for the remainder of the veggies.

The choice is all yours!

Day 12

Breakfast: Scrambled Eggs With Halloumi Cheese

Ingredients

5 to 6 eggs

3 ½ ounces diced Halloumi cheese

4 ½ ounces diced bacon

8 tablespoons each:

- Pitted olives
- Chopped fresh parsley

Pepper and Salt to taste

2 scallions

2 tablespoons olive oil

Instructions

1. Dice the bacon and cheese.

2. Over the stovetop, use the medium-high setting; pour the oil into a frying pan. Add the scallions, cheese, and bacon—sauté until browned.

3. Whip/Whisk the eggs, pepper, salt, and parsley in a mixing container.

4. Pour the mixture into the pan over the cheese and bacon.

5. Reduce the heat—toss in the olives and sauté for several minutes.

6. All Ready! You can enjoy this with or without a salad.

Yields: Two Servings

Lunch: Salmon with Spinach and Chili Tones

Ingredients

1 tablespoon chili paste

1 ½ Pounds Salmon (in pieces)

1 cup sour cream/mayonnaise

1 ¾ cup olive oil/butter

1 Pound fresh spinach

4 tablespoons grated parmesan cheese

Pepper and Salt

Instructions

1. Place the oven setting to 400°F/200°C. Use some cooking oil to coat a baking dish/pan.

2. Flavor the salmon with the pepper and salt. Place in the dish skin side down.

3. Blend the chili paste, sour cream/mayonnaise, and parmesan cheese and spread it on the filets.

4. Bake until the salmon is done—usually fifteen to twenty minutes.

5. In the meantime, sauté the spinach until it wilts using the oil/butter.

Yields: Four Servings

Dinner: Chicken Stuffed Avocado—Cajun Style

Ingredients

1 ½ cups cooked chicken (7.4 ounces or 210 g)

2 medium or 1 large avocados (10.6 ounces or 300 g)

2 tablespoons cream cheese/sour cream

2 tablespoons lemon juice (fresh)

¼ cup mayonnaise

½ teaspoon each: onion powder & garlic powder

¼ teaspoon each: salt and cayenne pepper

1 teaspoon each: paprika and dried thyme

Instructions

1. Shred the chicken into small pieces.

2. Blend all of the ingredients—saving the salt and lemon juice until last.

3. Leave one-half to one-inch of the avocado flesh—scoop the middle. Remove the seeds.

4. Cut the center/scooped pieces of avocado into small pieces and fill each of the halves with the mixture of chicken.

Yields: Two Servings

Serving Portion: Fat: 50.6 g; Carbs 16.4 g; Protein: 34.5 g

Day 13

Breakfast: Western Omelet

Ingredients

2 tablespoons sour cream/heavy whipping cream

6 eggs

Pepper and Salt

2 ounces butter

3 ½ ounces shredded cheese

5 ounces of ham

½ each:

- Finely chopped green bell peppers

- Finely chopped yellow onion

Instructions

1. Whisk the sour cream/cream and eggs until fluffy. Flavor with the pepper and salt. Add half of the cheese and combine.

2. Melt the butter on the stovetop on the medium heat setting. Sauté the peppers, onions, and ham for just a few minutes.

3. Pour the batter in and fry until the omelet is almost firm.

4. Lower the heat and Sprinkle the remainder of the cheese on top of your masterpiece. Fold the omelet right away.

Have a fresh green salad as a perfect brunch touch!

Yields: Two Servings

Lunch: Tortilla Ground Beef Salsa

Ingredients

1 ½ Pounds ground lamb/beef

8 to 12 low-carb tortilla breads

2 tablespoons olive oil

1 cup of water

Tex-Mex seasoning (see below)

 1 teaspoon salt

Shredded leafy greens

17 to 27 tablespoons shredded cheese

Salsa Ingredients

1 to 2 diced tomatoes

2 avocados

1 tablespoon olive oil

Juice of 1 lime

8 tablespoons fresh cilantro

Pepper and Salt

Tex-Mex Seasoning

2 tsp. each:

- Paprika powder
- Chili powder

1 to 2 tsp. garlic/onion powder

1 tsp. ground cumin

A pinch of cayenne pepper

Optional: 1 tsp. salt

Instructions

1. Prepare two batches of low-carb tortilla bread (see below).

2. Chop the cilantro. Take out the beef so it can become room temperature. Cold meats can have an effect on the cooking times, and it is more of a boil, not a fry.

3. On the stovetop, heat the oil using a large pan. Toss in the beef, and cook for around ten minutes.

4. Add the salt, water, and taco seasoning to the beef and simmer until most of the liquid has evaporated.

5. Meanwhile, prepare the salsa with all of the ingredients.

6. Serve on the tortilla bread with some shredded cheese along with the leafy greens.

Yields: Four Servings

Low-Carb Tortillas

Ingredients

2 egg whites

2 eggs

6 ounces cream cheese

1 tablespoon coconut flour

1 to 2 teaspoons ground psyllium husk powder

½ teaspoon salt

Instructions

1. Heat the oven to 400°F. Prepare two baking sheets with parchment paper.

2. Whip the eggs and whites until fluffy. Blend in the cream cheese and whisk until creamy.

3. Combine the coconut flour, psyllium powder, and salt in a small container. Add the flour mixture for the batter a spoon at a time.

4. Spread out the batter on the baking tins, spreading thin, about ¼-inch thick. You can make two rectangles or four to six circles.

5. Bake until the tortilla begins to brown around the edges, usually about five minutes (or so).

6. Serve with some of your *Tex-Mex Ground Beef and Salsa.*

Yields: Two Servings

Dinner: Fish Casserole with Mushrooms

Ingredients

1 Pound mushrooms

3 ¼ ounces butter

2 Tbsp. fresh parsley

1 t. salt

Pepper (to taste)

2 C. heavy whipping cream

2 tablespoons fresh parsley

2 to 3 Tbsp. Dijon mustard

1 ½ Pounds white fish (Ex. Cod)

½ Pound shredded cheese

1 1/3 pounds cauliflower/broccoli

3 ¼ ounces olive oil/butter

Instructions

1. Heat the oven to 350°F. Lightly grease a baking dish for the fish.

2. Slice the mushrooms into wedges. *Sauté* in a pan with the butter, pepper, salt, and other herbs.

3. Empty the mustard and cream into the mixture and reduce the heat. Simmer for five to ten minutes until the sauce thickens.

4. Flavor the fish with the pepper and salt and add it to the prepared container. Sprinkle with ¾ of the cheese. Pour the creamed mushroom mixture over it and the rest of the cheese as a topping.

5. Bake approximately thirty minutes if the fish are frozen (less if not). After 20 minutes, test the fish to see if it flakes apart easily. Remember, the fish will cook for several minutes after it is removed from the oven.

6. Prepare the cauliflower into small florets, removing the leaves and stalks. You can use the entire broccoli by cutting it into rods/lengthwise.

7. Boil the veggie of choice, drain and add some butter/olive oil.

8. Coarsely mash with a fork or wooden spoon; adding some pepper and salt, and serve with your fish.

Yields: Four Servings

Day 14

Breakfast: Blueberry Smoothie

Smoothie Ingredients

1 C. fresh or frozen blueberries

1 2/3 C. coconut milk

1 Tbsp. lemon juice

½ tsp. vanilla extract

Instructions

1. Put all of the ingredients into a tall beaker. Mix using a hand mixer.

2. Pour the lemon juice in for additional flavoring.

Notes: You can substitute 1 ¼ cups of Greek yogurt for a dairy option and adjust with a small amount of water if you are searching for more liquid consistency. Add 1 tablespoon of a healthy oil such as coconut for more satiety.

Yields: Two Servings

Lunch: Cheeseburger

Ingredients

7 ounces shredded cheese

1 ½ Pounds ground beef

2 teaspoons each:

- Onion powder

- Garlic powder

- Paprika

For Frying

2 tablespoons fresh oregano

Finely chopped butter

Salsa

2 scallions

2 tomatoes

1 avocado

Fresh Cilantro (to taste)

Salt

1 tablespoon olive oil

Toppings

- Lettuce
- Cooked bacon
- Dijon mustard
- Mayonnaise
- Pickled jalapenos
- Dill pickle

Instructions

1. Chop all of the salsa ingredients in a small container and set to the side.
2. Combine all of the seasonings and ½ of the cheese into the beef mixture.
3. Prepare four burgers and grill or pan fry to your liking—adding cheese at the end of the cooking cycle.
4. Serve on the bed of lettuce with some mustard and a dill pickle.

Yields: Four Servings

Dinner: Turkey with Cream Cheese Sauce

Ingredients

1 1/3 Pounds turkey breast

2 tablespoons butter

2 cups heavy whipping cream/sour cream

7 ounces cream cheese

Pepper and salt

1 tablespoon tamari soy sauce

6 ¾ tablespoons small capers

Instructions

1. Heat the oven to 350°F.

2. Sprinkle the turkey with pepper and salt for seasoning.

3. Add the butter to a frying pan. Sauté the turkey until golden. Place in the oven to finish cooking.

4. Using a small pan, combine the heavy cream/sour cream and cream cheese, bringing it to a boil; lower the heat and cook slowly for a few minutes.

5. On high heat in a small pan, use a small amount of butter or oil to fry the capers or enjoy them fresh.

6. When the turkey breast and veggies are done, add the sauce and capers on top of the turkey and serve along with some side dishes such as cauliflower or broccoli.

Yields: Four Servings

Chapter 3: Additional Breakfast Recipes

Chia Pudding

Ingredients

1 cup light coconut milk

¼ cup chia seeds

½ tablespoon light corn syrup

Instructions

1. Combine all of the ingredients in a small mason jar or bowl.

2. Refrigerate overnight. It is ready when the seeds have gelled, and the pudding is thick.

3. Add some nuts and fresh fruit and 'dive in.'

Cow-time Breakfast Skillet

Ingredients

2 medium diced sweet potatoes

1 Pound breakfast sausage

5 eggs

Handful of cilantro

1 diced avocado

Hot sauce

Optional: Raw cheese

Pepper and Salt

Instructions

1. Heat the oven to 400°F.

2. Use medium heat on the stovetop; place an iron or oven-safe skillet. Crumble and brown the sausage. Remove the sausage, cook the potatoes until crunchy, and reserve the grease.

3. Put the sausage back in the pan. Make some spaces in the 'wells' of the skillet, enough room for one egg. Crack the eggs into each of the wells.

4. Put the skillet into the preheated oven and bake enough for the eggs to set (about 5 minutes). Turn up the thermostat in the oven to the broil setting to let it broil the tops of the yolks with the crispy sweet potatoes.

5. Take the skillet out of the oven and cover it with some cilantro, avocado, and hot sauce.

Enjoy the tasty different flavors.

Cream Cheese Pancakes

Ingredients for the Pancakes

2 oz. (room temperature) cream cheese

2 organic eggs

½ teaspoon cinnamon

1 teaspoon granulated sugar substitute

Instructions

1. Place each of the pancake ingredients into a blender. Blend until creamy smooth; letting it rest for two minutes for the bubbles to settle back down.

2. Grease a pan with Pam spray or butter.

3. Pour about ¼ of the pancake batter into the hot pan; cooking for two minutes. Flip and continue cooking about one more minute.

4. Serve with berries or a sugar-free syrup of your choice.

Yields: Four Pancakes

Serving Size: 1 Batch: Carbs 2.5 g net; Fat 29; Protein 17 g; Calories 344

Dairy-Free Latte

Ingredients

2 Tbsp. coconut oil

1 2/3 C. hot water

2 eggs

1 tsp. ground ginger/pumpkin pie spice

Splash of vanilla extract

Instructions

1. Use a stick blender to combine all of the ingredients.

2. If you want to replace the spices; you can use 1 tablespoon of instant coffee or cocoa.

Enjoy for a quick boost!

Yields: Two Servings

Keto Sausage Patties

Ingredients

1 teaspoon maple extract

2 tablespoons granular Swerve Sweetener

½ teaspoon pepper

1 pound ground pork

2 tablespoons sage (chopped fresh)

1/8 teaspoon cayenne

1 teaspoon salt

¼ teaspoon garlic powder

Instructions

1. Combine each of the ingredients in a large mixing container.

2. Shape the patties to about a one-inch thickness.

3. The recipe will make eight equal patties.

4. Add a small amount of olive oil or a dab of butter to a pan over medium heat. For each side, allow three to four minutes.

Serving Portion: 2 patties: Carbs 1.4 g; Fat: 11 g; Protein: 21 g; Calories: 187

Keto Bacon

Use the Regular Oven

1. Preheat to 350 °F.

2. Put the bacon on a baking tray. Bake 20 to 25 minutes

3. Drain on a paper towel.

Use the Microwave

1. Put the bacon on paper towels in a single layer on a microwave-safe dish.

2. Use the high setting for four to six minutes.

Use the Skillet

1. Prepare the pan on the medium-low to medium.

2. Put the bacon into the pan single-layered.

3. Cook until the desired doneness is acquired.

Serving Portion: 2 slices: Fat: 19 g; Carbs 0.0 g; Protein: 7 g; Calories: 200

Mushroom Omelet

Ingredients

3 eggs

7/8 ounces shredded cheese

2 to 3 mushrooms

Optional: 1/5 of an onion

Pepper and salt to taste

For frying: 7/8 ounces butter

Instructions

1. Whisk the eggs with the pepper and salt, add the spices.

2. On the stovetop, use a frying pan to melt the butter. Pour in the eggs.

3. When the omelet begins to cook to firmness; sprinkle the mushrooms, cheese, and onion on top.

4. Ease the edges up using a spatula, and fold in half. Remove from the pan when golden brown.

If you are having brunch; add a crispy salad.

Yields: One serving

Chapter 4: Additional Lunch and Dinner Recipes

Deviled Eggs

With this tasty combination; it is hard to say breakfast or lunch; maybe brunch!

Ingredients

6 large eggs

¼ teaspoon yellow mustard

1 tablespoon mayonnaise

1 teaspoon paprika

Garnish: Parsley/salt/pepper

Optional

- ½ teaspoon cayenne pepper

- Several drops hot sauce

- 1 teaspoon cumin

Instructions

1. Slice the eggs lengthwise.

2. Mix the egg yolks with the rest of the ingredients.

3. Put the goodies inside the egg bed.

4. Sprinkle with condiments as desired.

Serving Portion: Fat: 20 g; Carbs 1 g; Protein: 19 g; Calories: 265

Ham and Apple Flatbread

Crust Ingredients

¾ cup almond flour

2 cups grated mozzarella cheese (part-skim)

2 tablespoons cream cheese

1/8 teaspoon dried thyme

½ teaspoon sea salt

Topping Ingredients

4 ounces sliced ham (low-carb)

½ small red onion

1 cup grated Mexican cheese

¼ medium apple

1/8 teaspoon dried thyme

Instructions

1. Remove the seeds and core from the apples. You can leave them unpeeled but will need to use a vegetable peeler to make the thin slices.

2. Heat the oven to 425°F.

3. Cut two pieces of parchment paper to fit into a 12-inch pizza pan (approximately two inches larger than the pan).

4. Use the high-heat setting and place a double boiler (water in the bottom pan), and bring the water to boiling. Lower the heat setting

and add the cream cheese, mozzarella cheese, salt, thyme, and almond flour to the top of the double boiler—stirring constantly.

5. When the cheese mixture resembles dough, place it on one of the pieces of parchment—and knead the dough until totally mixed.

6. Roll the dough into a ball—placing it at the center of the paper— place the second piece of paper over the top, and roll with a rolling pin (or a large glass).

7. Place the dough onto the pizza pan (leaving the paper connected).

8. Poke several holes in the dough and put into the preheated oven for approximately six to eight minutes.

9. When browned, remove it, and lower the setting of the oven to 350°F.

10. Arrange the cheese, apple slices, onion slices, and ham pieces.

11. Top off with the remainder (3/4 cup) of cheese.

12. Season with the ground pepper, salt, and thyme.

13. Place the finished product into the oven, baking until you see a golden brown crust.

14. Slide it from the parchment paper and cool two or three minutes before cutting.

Yields: Eight Slices

Tip: If you do not own a double boiler; you can substitute with a mixing dish over a pot of boiling water as a substitute.

Serving Portion: 1: Fat: 20 g; Carbs 5 g; Protein: 16 g; Calories: 255

Chicken Breast with Herb Butter

Ingredients for the Fried Chicken

4 Chicken Breasts

Pepper and Salt

1-ounce of olive oil/butter

Herb Butter Ingredients

1 clove garlic

1/3 Pound butter (room temperature)

1 tsp. lemon juice

½ tsp. each:

- garlic powder
- salt

4 Tbsp. fresh chopped parsley

Leafy Greens

½ Pound leafy greens (baby spinach for example)

Instructions

1. Take the butter out of the refrigerator for at least thirty to sixty minutes before you begin to prepare your meal.

2. Add all of the ingredients, including the butter, and blend thoroughly in a small container; set to the side.

3. Use the pepper and salt to flavor the chicken. Cook the chicken filets in a skillet using the butter over medium heat. To avoid dried out filets, lower the temperature the last few minutes.

4. Serve over a bed of greens with some melted herb butter over the top.

Yields: Four Servings

Low-Carbonara

Ingredients

2/3 Pounds diced Pancetta/bacon

1 ¼ cups heavy whipping cream

1 tablespoon butter

3 1/3 tablespoons mayonnaise

Fresh chopped parsley

Pepper and salt

2 Pounds zucchini

3 ½ ounces grated Parmesan cheese

4 egg yolks

Instructions

1. Empty the heavy cream into a saucepan, bringing it to a boil. Lower the burner and continue boiling until the juices are reduced by about a third.

2. Fry the bacon/pancetta; reserve the fat.

3. Combine the heavy cream, mayonnaise, pepper, and salt into the saucepan mixture.

4. Make 'zoodles' out of the zucchini using a potato peeler or spiralizer.

5. Add the zoodles to the warm sauce and serve with egg yolks, bacon, parsley, and freshly grated cheese.

6. Drizzle a bit of the bacon grease on top.

Yummy!

Yields: Four Servings

Pesto Chicken Casserole with Olives and Cheese

Ingredients

1 ½ Pounds chicken breasts/thighs

3 ½ ounces green or red pesto

8 tablespoons pitted olives

1 2/3 cups heavy whipping cream

½ Pound diced feta cheese

Pepper and Salt

1 finely chopped garlic clove

For Frying: Butter

For Serving

- Olive oil
- 1/3 Pound leafy greens
- Sea salt

Instructions

1. Heat the oven to 400°F.
2. Cut the chicken into pieces and flavor with the pepper and salt.
3. Place in a skillet with the butter, cooking until well done.
4. Combine the heavy cream and pesto.
5. Put the chicken pieces in the baking dish with the garlic, feta cheese, and olives, along with the pesto mix.
6. Bake for 20 to 30 minutes until the perfect color.

Enjoy with some green beans, sautéed asparagus, or another veggie of your choice.

Yields: Four Servings

Red Pesto Pork Chops

Ingredients

4 Pork chops

4 tablespoons red pesto

2 tablespoons olive oil/butter

6 tablespoons mayonnaise

Instructions

1. Thoroughly rub the chops with the pesto.

2. Fry on medium heat in a skillet with oil/butter for eight minutes. Reduce the heat and simmer four more minutes.

3. Serve with the pesto mayonnaise: 6 tablespoons of mayonnaise (+) 1 to 2 tablespoons pesto.

Serve with a large salad. You can also add a serving of cauliflower and broccoli with cheese.

Chapter 5: Snacks and Desserts for the Diet Plan

Keto Ginger Snap Cookies

Ingredients

¼ cup unsalted butter

1 large egg

2 C. almond flour

½ tsp. ground cinnamon

1 tsp. vanilla extract

1 C. sugar substitute/Erythritol (Swerve)

2 tsp. ground ginger

¼ tsp. each:

- Salt

- Ground cloves

- Nutmeg

Instructions

1. Set the oven to 350°F.

2. Combine the dry ingredients in a small dish.

3. Combine the remainder components to the dry mixture, and mix using a hand blender/mixer. (The dough will be crumbly and stiff.)

4. Measure out the dough for each cookie and flatten with a fork or your fingers.

5. Bake for approximately nine to eleven minutes or till they are browned.

Yields: 24 Cookies

Pumpkin Pudding

Ingredients

¼ cup pumpkin puree

1/3 cup granulated (Erythritol/Stevia)

½ tsp. pumpkin pie spices

1 tsp. xanthan gum

3 medium egg yolks

1 ½ cups whipping cream

1 tsp. vanilla extract

For the Cream Mixture

3 Tbsp. granulated stevia

1 cup whipping cream

½ tsp. vanilla extract

Instructions

1. Blend the pumpkin spice, xanthan gum, sweetener, and salt. Whip/whisk until the texture is smooth. Add the yolks, puree, and vanilla extract to the mixture; blend thoroughly.

2. Slowly pour in the whipping cream, after all of the cream is added. Using medium heat let the mixture come to a boil.

3. Continue the process for about 4 to 7 minutes, until thickened.

4. Place in the refrigerator in a container. Stir every ten minutes.

5. Meanwhile, in a medium dish, use a mixer to whip the one cup of whipping cream resulting in stiff peaks. Add the vanilla and sweetener; stir gently.

6. After the base pudding mixture has cooled; fold the whipped cream into the mix.

Scoop the pudding into small serving dishes and chill for a minimum of one to two hours.

Yields: Six Servings

No-Bake Cashew Coconut Bars

Ingredients

¼ cup maple syrup/sugar-free

1 cup almond flour

¼ cup melted butter

1 teaspoon cinnamon

½ cup cashews

A pinch of salt

1/4 cup shredded coconut

Instructions

1. Combine the flour and melted butter in a large mixing dish.

2. Add the maple syrup, cinnamon, salt, and coconut—blend well.

3. Use roasted or raw cashews. Chop them and add to the cashew-coconut bar dough. Blend well again.

4. Cover a cookie pan with parchment paper and spread the dough onto the paper in an even layer.

5. Place in the fridge for a minimum of two hours. Slice them and enjoy!

Yields: Eight Servings

Brownie Cheesecake

The Brownie Base Ingredients:

2 ounces chopped unsweetened chocolate

2 large eggs

½ cup butter

1/2 cup almond flour

1 pinch of salt

¼ cup cocoa powder

¾ cup granulated Erythritol/Swerve Sweetener

¼ cup pecans/walnuts (chopped)

¼ teaspoon vanilla

Cheesecake Filling Ingredients

2 large eggs

1 pound softened cream cheese

½ cup granulated sugar/Swerve sweetener

½ teaspoon vanilla extract

¼ cup heavy cream

Instructions

1. Butter a nine-inch springform pan; wrapping the bottom with foil.

2. Set the oven at 325°F.

3. Melt the chocolate and butter in a microwave-safe dish for 30 seconds.

4. Whisk the cocoa powder, almond flour, and salt in a small dish.

5. In a separate dish; whip the vanilla, eggs, and Swerve until smooth.

6. Blend the flour mixture and chocolate/butter mixture. Blend in the nuts.

7. Spread out in the prepared dish and bake for approximately 15 to 20 minutes.

8. Let it cool for about 20 to 25 minutes.

For the Filling

1. Reduce the oven setting to 300°F.

2. Blend the Swerve, the vanilla, cream, eggs, and cream cheese in a mixing container until everything is thoroughly mixed. Empty the filling ingredients into the crust and place it on a large cookie sheet.

3. Bake for about 35 to 45 minutes. The center should barely jiggle.

4. Loosen the edges with a knife.

5. Place them in the fridge for a minimum of three hours.

Yields: Ten Servings

Chocolate Soufflé

Ingredients

1 tablespoon butter

6 large egg whites

3 large egg yolks

5 ounces unsweetened chocolate

Note: The eggs work best at room temperature.

Instructions

1. Preset the oven to 375°F.

2. Use the butter to grease a soufflé dish.

3. Use a double boiler or a metal dish above a pan of boiling water to melt the chocolate. (Stir the mix constantly.)

4. Remove the dish and whip in the yolks until the mix hardens. Set it to the side.

5. Use a pinch of salt, whip/whisk the egg whites with an electric mixer on the highest setting.

6. Gradually, blend in the sugar/Lakanto. Continue until you see stiff peaks.

7. Stir in one cup of the egg whites into the chocolate combination folding gently using a silicone spatula. Pour the mixture into the soufflé dish.

8. Bake approximately twenty minutes. The center should still jiggle with the soufflé crusted and puffed on the top.

Serve this delicious treat right away.

Topping/Optional: Coconut whipped cream

Yields: Four Treats

Note: To make the soufflé rise evenly; use your thumb to remove the batter from the top of the dish.

Macaroon Keto Bombs

Your curiosity is wondering, "What is a bomb?" The reasoning is that this is good for you and is too delicious to pass by when you are craving a treat!

Ingredients

½ cup shredded coconut

¼ cup almond flour

2 tablespoons sugar substitute (Swerve)

3 egg whites

1 tablespoon each:

- Coconut oil
- Vanilla extract

Instructions

1. Set the oven at 400°F.

2. In a small container, combine the almond flour, coconut, and Swerve.

3. Use a small saucepan to melt the coconut oil. Add the vanilla extract.

4. *Note*: To mount the egg whites, place a medium dish in the freezer.

5. Add the oil to the flour mixture and blend well.

6. Break the egg whites in the cold dish and whip until stiff peaks are formed. Blend the egg whites into the flour mixture.

7. Spoon the mixture into a muffin cup or place them on a baking sheet.

8. Bake the macaroons for eight minutes or until you see browned edges.

9. Cool the bombs before you attempt to remove them from the pan.

Yields: Ten Servings

Conclusion

Thank for viewing your personal copy of the *Ketogenic Diet: Better Energy, Performance, and Natural Fuel to Good Health for the Smart*. Let's hope it was informative and able to provide you with all of the tools you need to achieve your goals as a better energy management specialist.

The next step is to test some of the recipes for yourself and discover what you have been missing since you have tried so many times unsuccessfully using other dieting methods. The recipes provided have been tested by qualified chefs who know the deal when it comes to energy performance.

Just remember, making advances towards a better lifestyle begins at the breakfast, lunch, and dinner table. You can supplement as you see fit once you have the knack of how the balance works.

Index for Recipes

Chapter 2: The 14-Day Plan

Day One

- Breakfast: Keto Scrambled Eggs

- Lunch: Tuna Cheese Melt (Low-Carbs)

- "Oopsie" Bread

- Dinner: Chicken Smothered in Creamy Onion Sauce

Day Two

- Breakfast: Mock Mc Griddle Casserole

- Brussels Sprouts with Hamburger Gratin

- Dinner: Squash and Sausage Casserole

Day Three

- Breakfast: Can't Beat it Porridge

- Lunch: Salad From a Jar

- Dinner: Ham and Cheese Stromboli

Day Four

- Breakfast: Frittata with Cheese and Tomatoes

- Lunch: Chicken—Broccoli—Zucchini Boats

- Dinner: Steak-Lovers Slow-Cooked Chili

Day 5

- Breakfast: Brownie Muffins

- Lunch: Bacon-Avocado-Goat Cheese Salad

- Dinner: Tenderloin Stuffed Keto Style

Day 6

- Breakfast: Sausage—Feta—Spinach Omelet

- Lunch: Pancakes with Cream-Cheese Topping

- Dinner: Skillet Style Sausage and Cabbage Melt

Day 7

- Breakfast: Tapas

- Lunch: Tofu—Bok-Choy Salad

- Dinner: Hamburger Stroganoff

Day 8

- Breakfast: Cheddar—Jalapeno Waffles

- Lunch: Salmon Tandoori with Cucumber Sauce

- Dinner: Ground Beef Stir Fry

Day 9

- Breakfast: Cheddar and Sage Waffles

- Lunch: Crispy Shrimp Salad on an Egg Wrap

- Dinner: Bacon Wrapped Meatloaf

Day 10

- Breakfast: Omelet Wrap with Avocado & Salmon

- Lunch: Tuna Avocado Melt

- Dinner: Hamburger Patties with Fried Cabbage

Day 11

- Breakfast: The Breadless Breakfast Sandwich

- Lunch: Thai Fish With Coconut & Curry

- Dinner: Keto Tacos or Nachos

Day 12

- Breakfast: Scrambled Eggs With Halloumi Cheese

- Lunch: Salmon with Spinach and Chili Tones

- Dinner: Chicken Stuffed Avocado—Cajun Style

Day 13

- Breakfast: Western Omelet

- Lunch: Tortilla Ground Beef Salsa

- Low-Carb Tortillas

- Dinner: Fish Casserole with Mushrooms

Day 14

- Breakfast: Blueberry Smoothie

- Lunch: Cheeseburger

- Dinner: Turkey with Cream Cheese Sauce

Chapter 3: Additional Breakfast Recipes

- Chia Pudding

- Cow-time Breakfast Skillet

- Cream Cheese Pancakes

- Dairy Free Latte

- Keto Sausage Patties

- Keto Bacon

- Mushroom Omelet

Chapter 4: Additional Lunch and Dinner Recipes

- Deviled Eggs

- Ham and Apple Flatbread

- Chicken Breast with Herb Butter

- Low-Carbonara

- Pesto Chicken Casserole with Olives and Cheese

- Red Pesto Pork Chops

Chapter 5: Snacks and Desserts for the Diet Plan

- Keto Ginger Snap Cookies

- Pumpkin Pudding

- No-Bake Cashew Coconut Bars

- Brownie Cheesecake

- Chocolate Soufflé

Macaroon Keto Bombs

PART 2

PART 2.1:

What Is Fasting and Why You Should Do It

Chapter 1: What Is Fasting?

Introduction to Fasting

Latest Research and Studies about Fasting

In a research published by the Springer Journal, it was found that fasting helps fight against obesity. The study, led by Kyoung Han Kim and Yun Hye Kim, was aimed at tracking the effects of fasting on fat cells. They put a group of mice into a four-month period of intermittent fasts, where the mice were fed for two days, followed by a day of fasting. In the end, the group of fasting mice was found to weigh less than the non-fasting mice, even though all of them had consumed exact quantities of food. The group of fasting mice had registered a drop in the fat buildup around fat cells. The explanation was that the fat had been converted into energy when glucose was insufficient. (www.sciencedaily.com/releases/ 2017/10/171017110041.htm)

In November 2017, Harvard researchers established that fasting can induce a long life, as well as minimize aging effects. It was found that fasting revitalizes mitochondria. Mitochondria are the organelles that act as body power plants. In this replenished state, mitochondria optimize physiological functions, in effect slowing down the aging process. Fasting also promotes low blood glucose levels, which improves skin clarity and boosts the immune system. (https://newatlas.com/fasting-increase-lifespan-mitochondria-harvard/52058/)

Sebastian Brandhorst, a researcher based at the University of Southern California, found out that fasting has a positive impact on brain health. Fasting induces low blood sugar levels, causing the liver to produce ketone bodies that pass on to the brain in place of sugars. Ketone bodies are much more stable and efficient energy sources than glucose. Researchers from the same university have posited that fasting minimizes chances of coming down with diabetes and other degenerative diseases. Moreover, they discovered that fasting induces low production of the IGF-1 hormone, which is a catalyst in aging and spread of disease. (https://www.cnbc.com/

2017/10/20/science-diet-fasting-may-be-more-important-than-just-eating-less.html)

Biological Effects of Fasting

- **Cleanses the body**

Our bodies harbor an endless count of toxins, and these toxins announce their presence through symptoms like low energy, infections, allergies, terrible moods, bloating, confusion, and so on.

Eliminating toxins from your body will do you a world of good in the sense that your body will upgrade and start functioning optimally. There are many ways to cleanse your body: hydrotherapy, meditation, organic diets, herbs, yoga, etc.

But one of the most effective ways of cleansing your body is through fasting. When you go on a fast, you allow the body to channel the energy that would have been used for digestion into flushing out toxins.

- **Improves heart health**

Studies show that people who undertake regular fasts are less likely to contract coronary infections. Fasting fights against obesity, and obesity is a recipe for heart disease. It purifies the blood too, in that sense augmenting the flow of blood around the body.

- **Improves the immune system**

Fasting rids the body of toxins and radicals, thus boosting the body's immune system and minimizes the chances of coming down with degenerative diseases like cancer. Fasting reduces inflammation as well.

- **Improves bowel movement**

One of the problems of consuming food on the regular is that the food sort of clogs up your stomach, causing indigestion. You might go for days without visiting the bathroom to perform number two. But when you fast, your body resources won't be bogged down by loads of undigested foods, and so your bowel movement will be seamless. Also, fasting promotes healthy gut bacteria.

- **Induces alertness**

When your stomach is full because of combined undigested foods (i.e., "garbage"), you are more likely to experience brain-fog. You won't have any concentration on the tasks at hand. You will just sit around and laze the hours away, belching and spitting. But when you fast, your mind will be clear so it will be easy to cultivate focus.

'Treating Fasting as a Lifestyle Choice

When you perform a simple Google search for the word "fasting," millions of results come up. Fasting is slowly becoming a mainstream subject. This is mostly because of the research-backed evidence that has been published by many reputable publications listing down the various benefits of fasting such as improved brain health, increased production of the human growth hormone, a stronger immune system, heart health, and weight loss—thus its appeal to health-conscious people as a catalyst for their health goals.

Taking up fasting as a lifestyle choice will see you go without food for anywhere from a couple of hours to days. But before you get into it, you'd do yourself a world of good to first obtain clearance from a physician, certifying that your body is ready, because not everyone is made for it. For instance, the symptoms of illnesses such as cancer may worsen after a long stretch of food deprivation. So people with degenerative diseases such as cancer should consider getting professional help or staying away altogether. Pregnant women, malnourished people, and children are advised to stay clear too.

The first thing you must do is to establish your fasting routine. For instance, you may choose to skip breakfast, making lunch your first meal of the day. Go at it with consistency. Also, you may decide to space your meals over some hours; so that when the set hours elapse, you reach your eating window, and then go back to fasting. The real challenge is staying committed. You will find that it will be difficult to break the cycle of eating that your body had been accustomed to, but when you persevere; your body will, of course, adjust to your new habit. If you decide to go for days without food, the results will be far pronounced, but please remember to hydrate your body constantly to flush out toxins.

Summary

Fasting is the willing abstinence from food over a period of time with the goal of improving your life. Conventionally, fasting has been tied to religious practices, but a new school of thought has emerged to proclaim the health benefits of fasting—particularly, weight loss. When you go into a fast, you create a caloric deficit, which triggers the body to convert its fat stores into energy. Numerous studies by mainstream health organizations have been done on fasting, and researchers have established that fasting has a host of advantages like improved motor skills, cognition, and moods. Some of the biological effects of fasting include improved bowel movement, immune system, and heart health. If you are starting out with fasting, you must create a routine and abide by it. Not everyone is fit to practice fasting. Some of the people advised to stay away from the practice include extremely sick people, pregnant women, the malnourished, and children. If you undertake a prolonged fast, you should hydrate your body constantly.

Chapter 2: Obesity and the Standard American Diet

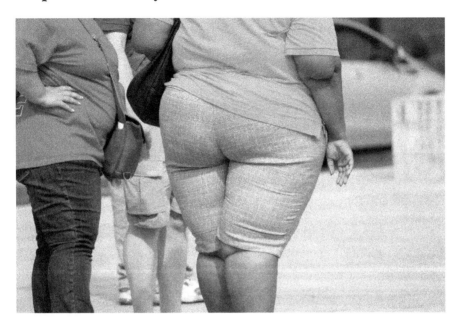

The Obesity Epidemic

We are killing ourselves with nothing more than a spoon and a fork. In 2017, obesity claimed more lives than car accidents, terrorism, and Alzheimer's combined. And the numbers are climbing at a jaw-dropping rate. Obesity has become a crisis that we cannot afford to ignore anymore.

You'd be mistaken to think that obesity is a crisis in first-world economies alone. Even developing nations are experiencing an upsurge of obese citizens. Here comes the big question: what is the **main** force behind this epidemic?

According to new research published in the New England Journal of Medicine, excessive caloric intake and lack of exercise are to blame.

Most American fast food chains have now become global. Fast foods, which are particularly calorie-laden, appeal to a lot of people across the world because of their low prices and taste. So, most people get hooked on the fast food diet and slowly begin the plunge into obesity.

The United States recognizes obesity as a health crisis and lawmakers have petitioned for tax increment on fast foods and sugary drinks, except that for a person who's addicted to fast foods, it would take a lot more than a price increase to discourage their food addiction. It would take a total lifestyle change.

Exercising alone won't help you; no matter how powerful your reps may be, or leg lifts or anything else you try in the gym, nothing can save you from a terrible diet.

And here's the complete shocker; the rate of childhood obesity has surpassed adulthood obesity; a terrible, terrible situation considering that childhood obesity almost always leads to heart complications in adult life.

Why Are We So Fat?

- **Poor food choices**

The number one reason why we are so fat is our poor choice of food. We eat too much of the wrong food, and most of it is not expended, so it becomes stored up as fat.

- **Bad genetics**

It's true that some people are genetically predisposed to gain more weight. Their genetics have wired them to convey abnormal hunger signals, so their bodies pressure them into consuming much more food.

- **Lack of strenuous activities**

Our modern-day lives involve only light physical tasks. Contrast that with the era of the dawn of humanity. Back then people would use up a lot of energy to perform physical activities and survive in unforgiving habitats. Most of the food they consumed would be actually utilized. But today, thanks to our technological advancement, we have been spared from taking part in laborious activities. This makes it hard to use up the energy from food, and the body opts to store it as fat.

- **Psychological issues**

Some of us react to bad moods by indulging in food—in particular, high-calorie fast foods—because the taste of fast foods appeals to our unstable emotions. When we fall in the habit of rewarding our bad moods or depression with binge eating, we unsuspectingly fall into the trap of food addiction, to the point of getting depressed when we fail to binge eat, kicking off our journey into obesity.

- **The endocrine system**

The thyroid's hormones play a critical role in the metabolic rate of a person. Ideally, a strong endocrine system means a high metabolic rate. And so, individuals who have a weakened endocrine system are much more likely to develop obesity.

The Problem with Calories

Calories are the basic units for quantifying the energy in the food we consume. A healthy man needs a daily dose of around 2500 calories to function optimally, and a woman needs 2000 calories.

This caloric target should be met through the consumption of various foods containing minerals, vitamins, antioxidants, fiber, and other important elements, and this is not hard at all to achieve if you adhere to the old-fashioned "traditional diet."

But the challenge is that nowadays, we have many foods with a high caloric count, and yet they hardly fill us up! For instance, fries, milkshake, and a burger make up nearly 2000 calories! You can see how easy it'd be to surpass the caloric limit by indulging in fast food.

When we consume more calories than we burn, our bodies store up the excess calories as fat, and as this process repeats itself over time, the fat has a compounding effect that leads to weight gain.

The only way to make your weight stable is through balancing out the energy you consume with the energy you expend. But for someone who suffers from obesity, if they'd like to have a normal weight, they must create a caloric deficit, and fasting is the surefire practice of creating such a deficit.

Besides checking your caloric intake, you might also consider improving your endocrine system and the efficiency of both your kidney and liver, because they have a direct impact on how the body burns calories. When you buy food products, always find out their caloric count to assess how well they'll fit within your daily caloric needs.

The American Diet

In a 2016 lifestyle survey, most Americans admitted that it is not easy to keep their diet clean and healthy. This isn't surprising, especially when you consider the fact that the average American consumes more than 20 pounds of sweeteners each year. The over-emphasis of sugar and fat in the American diet is the leading cause of obesity in Americans. Illnesses triggered by obesity long started marching into our homes. What we have now is a crisis. But let's find out the exact types of foods that Americans like to feast on (we are big on consuming, it's no secret).

As a melting point of cultures drawn from various parts of the world, it's kind of difficult to say exactly what the all-American favorite foods are. But the United States Department of Agriculture might shine some light on this. It listed down desserts, bread, chicken, soda, and alcohol, as the top five sources of calories among Americans. As you can see, the sugar intake is impossibly high. Interestingly, the US Department of Agriculture also noted that Americans aren't big on fruits.

Pizza may qualify as the all-time favorite snack of America, followed closely by burgers and other fast food. There is a reason why most fast food restaurants are successful in America and throughout the world.

It has also been established that the average American drinks about a gallon of soda every week. Even drinks that are supposed to have a low-calorie count end up being calorie-bombs because of the doctoring that takes place. For instance, black coffee is low on calorie, but not so if it has milk and ice cream and sugar all over it.

Summary

The first-world economies are not alone in facing the crisis of obesity. It has emerged that people in poor countries are battling obesity too. Obesity-related deaths are on the rise. In 2017, the figures were especially shocking, for they'd surpassed the death count of terrorist attacks, accidents, and Alzheimer's combined. One of the corrective measures that the US government is considering to undertake is tax increment on sugars. The chief reason why we are so fat is our poor diets. Our foods are laden with sugars and fats, and it doesn't help that our lifestyles allow us to expend only a small amount of energy, which leads to fat accumulation and consequent weight gain. The average man requires around 2500 calories for his body to act optimally whereas the average woman requires 2000 calories. The top five daily sources of calories for Americans include desserts, bread, chicken, soda, and alcohol.

Chapter 3: Benefits of Fasting

- **Improved Insulin Sensitivity**

Insulin sensitivity refers to how positively or negatively your body cells respond to insulin. If you have a high insulin sensitivity, you will need less amount of insulin to convert the sugars in your blood into energy, whereas someone with low insulin sensitivity would need a significantly larger amount of insulin.

Low insulin sensitivity is characterized by increased blood sugar levels. In other words, the insulin produced by the body is underutilized when converting sugars into energy. Low insulin sensitivity may make you vulnerable to ailments such as cancer, heart disease, type 2 diabetes, stroke, and dementia.

Ailments and bad moods are the general causes of low insulin sensitivity. However, high insulin sensitivity is restored once the ailments and bad moods are over.

Fasting is shown to have a positive effect on insulin sensitivity, enhancing your body to use small amounts of insulin to convert blood sugar into energy.

Improved insulin sensitivity has a great impact on health: leveling up physiological functions and fighting off common symptoms of ailments like lightheadedness and lethargy.

To increase insulin sensitivity, here are some of the best practices: perform physical activities, lose weight, consume foods that are high in fiber and low in Glycemic load, improve your moods and alleviate depressed feelings, and finally, make sure to improve the quality of your sleep.

The rate of insulin sensitivity is also heavily dependent on lifestyle changes. For instance, if you take up sports and exercise, insulin sensitivity goes up, but if you become lazy and inactive, it goes down.

- **Increased Leptin Sensitivity**

Leptin is the hormone that determines whether you're experiencing hunger or full. This hormone plays a critical role in weight loss and health management, and if your body grows insensitive to it, you become susceptible to some ailments. Understanding the role of leptin in your body is critical as it goes into helping you improve your health regimen.

Whenever this hormone is secreted by the fat cells, the brain takes notice, and it tries to determine whether you are in need of food or are actually full. Leptin needs to work as normally as possible else you will receive an inaccurate signal that will cause you to either overfeed or starve yourself.

Low leptin sensitivity induces obesity. This condition is normally witnessed in people with high levels of insulin. The excessive sugars in blood are carried off by insulin into fat cells, but when there is an insulin overload, a communication crash is triggered between fat cells and the brain. This condition induces low leptin sensitivity. When this happens, your brain is unable to tell the exact amount of leptin in your blood, and as such it misleads you. Low leptin sensitivity causes the brain to continue sending out the hunger signal even after you are full. This causes you to eat more than you should and, given time, leads to chronic weight gain.

Fasting has been shown to increase leptin sensitivity, a state that allows the brain to be precise in determining blood leptin quantities, and ensures that the accurate signal is transmitted to control your eating habits.

- **Normalized Ghrelin Levels**

Known as the "hunger hormone," ghrelin is instrumental in regulating both appetite and the rate of energy distribution into body cells.

Increased levels of ghrelin cause the brain to trigger hunger pangs and secrete gastric acids as the body anticipates you to consume food.

It is also important to note that both ghrelin and leptin receptors are located on the same group of brain cells, even though these hormones play contrasting roles, i.e., ghrelin being the hunger hormone, and leptin the satiety hormone.

The primary role of ghrelin is to increase appetite and see to it that the body has a larger fat reservoir. So, high ghrelin levels in your blood will result in you wanting to eat more food and, in some cases, particular foods like cake or fries or chocolate.

People who have low ghrelin levels will not eat enough amounts of food and are thus vulnerable to diseases caused by underfeeding. As a corrective measure, such people should receive shots of ghrelin to restore accurate hunger signals in their bodies.

Studies show that obese people suffer from a disconnection between their brains and ghrelin cells, so the blood ghrelin levels go through the roof, which makes these people be in a state of perpetual hunger. So, these obese people respond to their hunger pangs by indulging in their foods of choice, and thus the chronic weight gain becomes hard to manage.

It has been proven that fasting has a positive effect on ghrelin levels. Fasting streamlines the faulty communication between the brain receptors and ghrelin cells. When this is corrected, the brain starts to send out accurate hunger signals, discouraging you from eating more than you should.

- **Increased Lifespan And Slow Aging**

A study by Harvard researchers demonstrated that intermittent fasting led to an increased lifespan and the slowing down of the aging process. These findings were largely hinged on the cell-replenishing effects of fasting and flushing out of toxins.

The average person puts their digestive system under constant load because they're only a short moment away from their next meal. And given the fact that most foods are bacteria-laden, the immune system becomes strained with all the wars that it must be involved in. This makes the body cells prone to accelerated demise. But what happens when you go on a fast?

The energy that would have previously gone into digesting food is used to flush out toxins from the body instead. Also, it has been observed that body cells are strengthened during a fast, which makes physiological functions a bit more robust.

Fasting also enhances the creation of new neural pathways and regeneration of brain cells. This goes towards optimizing the functions of your brain. And, as we know, an energetic brain makes for a "youthful" life.

When you are on a fast, the blood sugar levels are generally down. The skin responds favorably to low blood sugar levels by improving elasticity and keeping wrinkles at bay. A high blood sugar level is notorious for making you ashy and wrinkly.

Fasting may increase your lifespan even from an indirect perspective. For instance, fasting may develop your sense of self-control, improve your discipline, and even increase your creativity. These immaterial resources are very necessary for surviving in the real world.

- **Improved Brain Function**

Fasting triggers the body to destroy its weak cells in a process known as autophagy. One of the main benefits of autophagy is reducing inflammation. Also, autophagy makes way for new and healthy body cells. Autophagy promotes neurogenesis, which is the creation of new brain cells.

Fasting allows the body to deplete the sugars in the blood, and since the body must continue to operate lest it shuts down, the body turns to an alternative energy source: fats. Through the aid of the liver, ketone bodies are produced to supply energy to the brain. Ketone bodies are a much cleaner and reliable source of energy than carbohydrates. Ketone bodies are known to tone down the effects of inflammatory diseases like arthritis.

Fasting promotes high insulin sensitivity. In this way, the body uses less insulin to convert sugars into energy. High insulin sensitivity means that the body will send out accurate signals when it comes to informing the host of either hunger or satiation.

Fasting enhances the production of BDNF (Brain-Derived Neurotrophic Factor), which a plays a critical part in improving neuroplasticity. And thus more resources are committed to the functions of the brain. BDNF is responsible for augmenting areas like memory, learning, and emotions.

Fasting supercharges your mind. It does so through facilitating the creation of new mitochondria. And since mitochondria are the power plants of our bodies, the energy output goes up. This increase in energy and resources causes the brain to function at a much higher level and yields perfect results.

- **Improved Strength And Agility**

When you think of a person that is considered strong and agile, your mind might conceive a well-muscled individual with veins bulging out their neck. Strength and agility come down to practice and more practice. The easiest way to develop agility and strength is obviously through physical training and sticking to a routine until your body adapts.

You must practice every day to be as strong and agile as you'd want to be. Also, you must take particular care over your dietary habits. Professional athletes stick to a diet that has been approved by their doctors for a reason. When it comes to developing strength and agility, nothing matches the combination of exercise and a flawless diet.

But besides fulfilling these two requirements, fasting, too, has its place. Did you know that you can amplify your strength and agility through fasting?

Fasting provokes the body to secrete the Human Growth Hormone. This hormone enhances organ development and even muscle growth. So when you fast, the HGH hormone might be secreted, and it will amplify the effects of your exercise and diet regimen, making you many times stronger and agile.

Fasting will promote the renewal of your body cells and thus lessen the effects of inflammation. When you perform physical exercises, you're basically injuring and damaging your body cells. So, when you fast, you'll allow your body to destroy its weak cells, and make room for new body cells through biogenesis.

Additionally, fasting will go a long way toward improving your motor skills, making you walk with the grace of a cat, with your body parts flexible.

- **Improved Immune System**

The immune system is responsible for defending your body against organisms that are disease vectors. When a foreign organism enters your body, and the body considers it harmful, the immune system immediately comes into action.

Some of the methods suggested for improving the immune system include having a balanced diet, quality sleep, improving your mental health, and taking physical exercises.

Fasting is an understated method of boosting your immune system.

In a research conducted by scientists at the University of Southern California, it emerged that fasting enhanced the rejuvenation of the immune system. Specifically, new white blood cells were formed, strengthening the body's defense system.

The regeneration of the immune system is especially beneficial to people who have a weak body defense mechanism—namely, the elderly, and the sick. This could probably be the reason why an animal in the wild responds to illness by abstaining from food.

In the same study, it was shown that there is a direct correlation between fasting and diminished radical elements in the body. Cell biogenesis was responsible for eradicating inflammation. And moreover, a replenished immune system discouraged the growth of cancer cells.

Depending on how long you observe a fast, the body will, at one point, run out of sugars, and then it will turn to your fat reservoirs to provide energy for its many physiological functions. Fats make for a much cleaner and stable and resourceful energy source than sugars ever will.

So, relying on this fat-energy, the immune system tends to function at a most optimal level.

- **Optimized Physiological Functions**

These are some of the body's physiological functions: sweating, bowel movement, temperature regulation, urinating, and stimuli response.

In a healthy person, all physiological functions should be seamless, but that cannot be said for most of us because our lifestyles get in the way.

So, the next time you rush to the bathroom intending to take a number two only to wind up spending half an hour there, you might want to take a close look at what you are eating.

Fasting is a great method of optimizing your physiological functions. When you observe a normal eating schedule, your body is under constant strain to keep digesting food—a resource-intensive process. But when you go on a fast, the energy that would have been used for digesting food will now be channeled into other critical functions. For instance, the body may now start ridding itself of radicals that promote indigestion, or amp up the blood circulation system, or even devote energy toward enhancing mental clarity, with the result being optimized physiological functions.

With more resources freed up from the strain of digestion, physiological processes will continue seamlessly, and once the glycogen in the blood is over, the body will continue to power physiological functions with energy acquired from fat cells.

The cellular repair benefits attached to fasting enables your body to perform its functions way better. Fasting reduces oxidative stress, which is a key accelerator of aging. In this way, fasting helps restore the youthfulness of your body cells, and the cells are very much optimized for performance.

- **Improved Cardiovascular Health**

When we talk about cardiovascular health, we are essentially talking about the state of the heart, and specifically, its performance in blood circulation.

Factors that improve the condition of your heart include a balanced diet, improved emotional and mental state, quality sleep, and living in a good environment. When cardiovascular health is compromised, it might lead to fatal consequences.

Researchers have long established that fasting improves cardiovascular health.

One of the outcomes of fasting is cholesterol reduction. The lesser cholesterol you have in your blood, the more seamless the movement of blood through your body. Complications are minimal or nonexistent. Thus your heart will be in a great condition.

Fasting also plays a critical role in toning down diabetes. The average diabetic tends to have low insulin sensitivity. For that reason, they need more insulin than is necessary to convert sugars into energy. It puts a strain on body organs and especially the pancreas. This might cause a trickle-down complication that goes back to the heart.

When the body enters fasting mode, it starts using up the stored energy to fulfill other important physiological functions such as blood circulation, in this way boosting the effectiveness of the heart.

Fasting helps you tap into your "higher state." The effects of matured spiritual energy and peaceful inner self cannot be gainsaid. Someone who's at peace with both himself and the universe is bound to develop a very healthy heart, as opposed to one who's constantly bitter, and one who feels as though he's drowning in a bottomless pit.

- **Low Blood Pressure**

People who have a high blood pressure are at risk of damaging not only their heart but their arteries too. When the pressure of the blood flowing in your arteries is high over a long period of time, it is bound to damage the cells of your arteries, and in the worst case scenario, it might trigger a rupture, and cause internal bleeding. High blood pressure puts you at risk of heart failure. Your heart might overwork itself and slowly start wearing out, eventually grinding to a halt.

In people with high blood pressure, a bigger-than-normal left heart is common, and the explanation is that their left heart struggles to maintain the cardiovascular output. So it starts bulking up and eventually creates a disrupting effect on your paired organ. Another risk associated with high blood pressure is coronary disease. This ailment causes your arteries to thin out to the point that it becomes a struggle for blood to flow into your heart. The dangers of coronary disease include arrhythmia, heart failure, and chest pain.

I started by mentioning the risks of high blood pressure because observing a fast normalizes your blood pressure. With a normal blood pressure, you can reverse these risks. Also, normal blood pressure improves the sensitivity of various hormones like ghrelin and leptin, eliminating the communication gap between brain receptors and body cells.

The low blood pressure induced by fasting causes you to have improved motor skills. It is common to hear people admit that fasting makes them feel light and flexible.

- **Decreased Inflammation**

Inflammation is an indication that the body is fighting against an infectious organism. It causes the affected parts to appear red and swollen.

Many diseases that plague us today are rooted in inflammation, and by the look of things, inflammation will be stuck with us for longer than we imagine.

The role of inflammation in mental health cannot be understated. Inflammation is to blame for bad moods, depression, and social anxiety.

The good news though is that fasting can reduce inflammation. Fasting has been shown to be effective in treating mental problems that are rooted in inflammation and as well as safeguarding neural pathways.

Individuals who have incorporated fasting into their lives are much less likely to suffer breakdowns and bad moods than people who don't fast at all.

Asthma, a lung infection, also has an inflammatory background. What's interesting is that fasting alleviates the symptoms of asthma.

The level of hormone sensitivity determines absorption rates of various elements into body cells. For instance, low insulin sensitivity worsens the rate of conversion of sugar into energy. Fasting improves insulin sensitivity, and thus more sugars can be converted into energy.

Fasting enhances the brain to form new pathways when new information is discovered. In this way, your memory power receives a boost, and you are better placed to handle stress and bad thoughts.

Fasting is very efficient in alleviating gut inflammation. Constant fasting promotes healthy gut flora which makes for great bowel movements.

Fasting is a great means of reducing heart inflammation, too. It does so through stabilizing blood pressure and fighting off radical elements.

- **Improved Skin Care**

Most of us are very self-conscious about how we look to the world. Bad skin, acne, and other skin ailments can be a real bother. Fasting has numerous benefits when it comes to improving your skin health, and it is said that fasting bestows a glow on your face. Experts claim that skin ailments develop as a result of terrible stomach environments and that there is a correlation between gut health and skin quality. Fasting promotes the development of gut flora. In this way, your gut health is improved, resulting in improved skin.

When you are on a fast and are taking water, you will eliminate toxins from your body. The condition of your skin improves because the skin cells are free of harmful substances. Many people who previously suffered from a bad skin condition and had tried almost every treatment with no success have admitted that fasting was the only thing that worked.

Another benefit of fasting is that it slows down the aging process. The water consumed during the fast goes to flush out toxins, consequently reducing the effects of old age on your skin. Fasting also promotes low blood sugar. Low blood sugar promotes optimized physiological processes and, as a result, toning down the effects of aging.

When you go on a fast, the body allocates energy to areas that might have previously been overlooked. So, your bad skin condition may be treated with the stored up energy, and considering that the energy produced from fat is more stable and resourceful; your skin health will improve.

- **Autophagy**

This is the process whereby the body rids itself of weakened and damaged cells. Autophagy is triggered by dry fasting. The body simply "eats" the weakened cells to provide water to the healthy cells. Eliminated cells are usually weak and damaged. And their absence creates room for new cells that are obviously going to be powerful.

Autophagy has been shown to have many benefits, and they include:

- **Slowing down aging effects**

The formation of wrinkles and body deterioration are some of the effects of aging. However, thanks to autophagy, these effects can be reversed, since the body will destroy its old and weakened cells and replace them with new cells.

- ## Reducing inflammation

Inflammation is responsible for many diseases affecting us today, but thanks to autophagy, the cells that have been affected by inflammation are consumed, giving room for new cells.

- ## Conserving energy

Autophagy elevates the body into a state of energy conservation. In this way, your body can utilize resources in a most careful manner.

- ## Fighting infections

The destruction of old and weak body cells creates room for fresh and powerful body cells. In that vein, old and weakened white blood cells are destroyed, and then new powerful white blood cells are formed. These new white new blood cells fortify the immune system.

- ## Improving motor skills

Autophagy plays a critical role in improving the motor skills of an individual. This goes toward boosting the strength and agility of a person. Energy drawn from the weak and damaged cells is way more resourceful than the energy drawn from sugars.

Summary

There are numerous benefits attached to fasting. One of them is increased insulin sensitivity. When the insulin sensitivity goes up, insulin resistance drops, and the body is now able to use less insulin to convert sugars into energy. Another benefit of fasting is improved leptin sensitivity. The leptin hormone is known as the satiation hormone, and it is responsible for alerting you when you are full. An improved ghrelin level is another benefit of fasting. The ghrelin hormone is known as the hunger hormone. It induces hunger pangs so that you may feed. Fasting lengthens your existence. This is largely because of neuroregeneration of cells and flushing out toxins. Fasting improves brain function, strengthens your body and boosts agility, strengthens your immune system, optimizes your physiological functions, improves cardiovascular health, lowers blood pressure, reduces inflammation, improves your skin, and promotes autophagy. As researchers carry out new experiments, more benefits of fasting are being uncovered.

Chapter 4: Myths and Dangers of Fasting

Long-Held Myths and Misconceptions about Fasting

Fasting has gained widespread acceptance across the world. More people who are seeking to improve their health through alternative means are turning to fasting. As you might expect, the field has been marred with conspiracies, lies, half-truths, and outright ignorance. Some of the long-held myths and misconceptions about fasting include:

Fasting makes you overeat. This myth hinges on the idea that after observing a fast, an individual is bound to be so hungry that they will consume more food to compensate for the period they'd abstained from food.

The brain requires a steady supply of sugars. Some people say that the brain cannot operate normally in the absence of sugars. These people believe that the brain uses sugars alone to power its activities and any other source of energy would not be compatible. So when you fast, you'd be risking shutting down your brain functions.

Skipping breakfast will make you fat. Some people seem to treat breakfast as though it were an unexplained mystery of the Earth. They say breakfast is special. Anyone who misses breakfast cannot possibly have a healthy life. They say that if you skip breakfast, you will be under a heavy spell of cravings, and finally give in to unhealthy foods.

Fasting promotes eating disorders. Some people seem to think that fasting is the stepping stone for disorders like bulimia and anorexia. They complain that once you see the effects of fasting, you might want to "amplify" the effects which might make you susceptible to an eating disorder like anorexia.

Busting Myths Associated with Fasting

Fasting will make you overeat. This is partly true. However, it is important to note that most people fall into the temptation of overeating because of their lack of discipline and not necessarily because of unrealistic demands of fasting. If you're fasting the proper way, no temptation is big enough to lead you astray, and after all, the temptation exists to test whether you're really disciplined.

The brain requires a steady supply of sugars. This myth perpetuates the notion that we should consume carbohydrates every now and again to keep the brain in working condition. Also, this myth suggests that the brain can only use energy derived from sugars and not energy derived from fats. When you go on a fast, and your body uses up all the glycogen, your liver produces ketone bodies that are passed on to your brain to act as an energy source.

Skipping breakfast will make you fat. There is nothing special about breakfast. You can decide to skip breakfast and adhere to your schedule and be able to get desired results. It's true that skipping breakfast will cause you to be tempted by cravings, but you're not supposed to give in, and in that case, you become the problem. Skipping breakfast will not make you fat. What will make you fat is you pouring more calories into your body than you will spend.

Fasting promotes eating disorders. If you have a goal in mind, you are supposed to stay focused on that goal. The idea that an individual would plunge into the world of eating disorders simply because they want to amplify the results of fasting sounds like weakness on the part of the individual and not a fault of the practice itself.

Dangers of Fasting

Just as with most things in life, there's both a positive and negative side to fasting. Most of these problems are amplified in people who either fast in the wrong way or people who clearly shouldn't be fasting.

So let's explore some of the risks that are attached to fasting.

- **Dehydration**

Chances are, you will suffer dehydration while observing a fast, and drinking regular cups of water won't make the situation any better. Well, this is because most of your water intake comes from the foods that you consume daily. When dehydration kicks in, you are bound to experience nausea, headaches, constipation, and dizziness.

- **Orthostatic Hypotension**

This is common in people who drink water during their fasts. Orthostatic Hypotension causes your body to react unfavorably when you move around. For instance, when you stand on your feet and walk around, you might experience dizziness and feel as though you're at the verge of blowing up into smithereens. Other symptoms include temporary mental blindness, lightheadedness, and vision problems. These symptoms make it hard for you to function in activities that demand precision and focus, e.g., driving.

- **Worsened medical conditions**

People who fast while they are sick put themselves at risk of worsening their condition. The fast may amplify the symptoms of their diseases. People with the following ailments should first seek doctor's approval before getting into fasting: gout, type 2 diabetes, chronic kidney disease, eating disorders, and heartburn.

- **Increased stress**

The habit of skipping meals might lead to increased stress. The body might respond to hunger by increasing the hormone cortisol which is responsible for high-stress levels. And when you are in a stressed mental state, it becomes difficult to function in your day to day life.

Summary

Although fasting has a lot of benefits, there is a dark side to it too, but the negative effects can be minimized or eliminated altogether when a professional is involved. Dehydration is one of the negative effects. Besides providing nutrients to the body, food is also an important source of water. So when you fail to correct this gap by drinking a lot more water, your body will fall into a state of dehydration. Orthostatic hypotension is another danger. This illness makes you feel dizzy and lightheaded, and so it makes it difficult for you to function in an activity that demands your focus and stamina. Fasting may amplify the symptoms of your disease depending on your age and the stage of your disease. For instance, people who suffer from illnesses like gout, diabetes, eating disorders, and heartburn should first seek the doctor's approval before going on a fast. Moreover, fasting may lead to an increase in stress levels.

Chapter 5: Safety, Side Effects, and Warning

The Safest and Enlightened Way of Fasting

As the subject of fasting becomes popular, more people are stating their opinions on it, and as you might expect, some people are for it, and others are against it.

The best approach toward fasting is not set in stone, but it is rather determined by factors such as your age and health status.

Before you get into fasting, there are some critical balances you need to consider first. One of them is your experience. If you have never attempted a fast before, then it is a bad idea to go straight into a 48-hour fast, because you are likely to water down the effects. As a beginner, you must always start with lighter fasts and build your way up into extended fasts. You could begin by skipping one meal, then two meals, and finally the whole day.

Another important metric when it comes to determining the appropriate space between your eating windows is your health status. For instance, you cannot be a sufferer of late-stage malaria and yet go on a fast, because it might create a multiplying effect on your symptoms. People who are malnourished or have eating disorders might want to find other ways of improving their health apart from fasting.

An essential thing to note is that we are not all alike. My body's response to a fast is not going to be the exact response of yours. Knowing this, always listen to your body. Sometimes, a water-fast might trigger a throat infection and make your throat swollen. In such a situation, it would be prudent to suspend the fast and take care of your throat, as opposed to sticking to your guns.

Side Effects of Fasting

Fasting might upset the physiological functions of a body. This explains the side effects that crop up when you go on a fast. It is also important to note that most of these side effects subside as your body grows accustomed to the fast.

- **Cravings**

Top on the list is cravings. When you go on a fast, the immediate response by the body is to elevate the "hunger hormone" and so, you will start craving for sweet unhealthy foods. If you are not the disciplined type, this is a huge pitfall that could negate the effects of your fast.

- **Headaches**

Headaches, too, are a side effect of fasting. Most people who are new to fasting are bound to experience a headache. One of the explanations for headaches is that it is the brain's response to a shift from relying on carbohydrates to ketone bodies as the alternative energy source. Regular consumption of water might mitigate the headache or eliminate it altogether.

- **Low energy**

Another side effect is low energy. When you fast, the body might interpret it as starving, and its first response will be conserving energy. So, there will be less energy for physiological functions. In this way, you will start feeling less energetic than before.

- **Irritability**

Irritability is also a side effect. Studies show that people who are new to fasting are bound to have foul moods as their body increases stress hormones and hunger hormones. However, if they can persist, the irritability will eventually go away, and make room for a happy mood as the body switches to its fat stores for energy.

Types of People That Should Not Fast

The ideal person to go on a fast is a healthy person. People with certain medical conditions may still go on a fast, but it is always prudent to seek the guidance of a medical professional. We have previously stated that fasting strengthens the immune system. So is it contradicting to discourage fasting when one is sick? No! You may fast but preferably under the instruction and supervision of a medical professional. However, there are cases when it is inappropriate to fast.

Infants and children. Putting kids on a fast is just wrong. Their bodies are not fully developed yet to withstand periods of hunger. Fasting would do them more damage than good. For instance, it might mess with their metabolism and have a negative impact on their growth curve.

Hypoglycemics. People with hypoglycemia have extremely low levels of blood sugar. Their bodies need a constant stream of sugars to sustain normal functions lest severe illnesses take reign. For that reason, hypoglycemics should not fast.

Pregnant and nursing women. These women need a lot of energy because their young ones are dependent on them. So, pregnant women and nursing women are encouraged to keep their blood sugar steady.

The malnourished. People who are underweight and malnourished should stay away from fasting. To start with, their bodies don't have sufficient fat. So, when they go on a fast, their body will destroy its cells in search of nutrients. Over time, the results could be fatal.

People with heartburn. People who experience severe heartburn should not fast. This is because heartburn is a very distressing thing and there is no guarantee it will subside even when your body adapts to fasting. So, it is better to stay clear.

Impaired immune system. Fasting may have the ability to renew the strength and utility of your immune system. But when we are talking about an impaired immune system where most of the white blood cells are hanging on a thin blade, then fasting cannot be of help. Such a person would be better off sticking to a healthy diet.

Other classes of people that shouldn't fast include those recovering from surgeries, people with eating disorders, depressed souls, and people with extreme heart disease.

Summary

For purposes of safety, always ensure that your body is prepared to withstand the effects of fasting. You may prepare by evaluating your health status, experience, and developing a great sense of self-awareness. Fasting may have its numerous benefits, but there is also a negative side to it because fasting comes with unpleasant side effects. The good thing though is that most of these side effects tend to subside once the body grows accustomed to your fasting routine. One of the side effects of fasting is getting a headache. A headache is triggered by the brain's adjustment from relying on carbohydrates as an energy source and switching to ketone bodies. It may be mitigated through constant consumption of water. Another side effect is cravings. Your body makes you want to eat fast foods very badly. Fasting may also make you irritable, but it is for only a short time and then a happy mood sets in. Fasting also makes you feel less energetic, which can be uninspiring. These are some of the people that shouldn't fast: hypoglycemics, infants, children, pregnant women, nursing women, the malnourished, people with extreme ailments, and those recovering from surgeries.

PART 2.2:

Types of Fasting and How to Fast

Chapter 6: Intermittent Fasting

What Is Intermittent Fasting?

Nowadays, intermittent fasting is one of the most talked about practices in health improvement domains. Basically, intermittent fasting is about creating a routine where you eat only after a set period of time. Intermittent fasting has been shown to have numerous benefits such as improving motor skills, developing willpower, and brain functions. Most people are turning to the practice to achieve their health goals—specifically, weight loss.

The most common way of performing an intermittent fast is by skipping meals. In the beginning, you may decide to skip one of the main meals, and when your body adapts to two meals a day, you may then elevate to just one meal per day. During the fast, you are not supposed to partake of any food, but it is okay to drink water and other low-calorie drinks like black coffee or black tea.

Intermittent fasting allows you to indulge in the foods of your choice, but there's emphasis on avoiding foods that are traditionally bad for your health. The main thing is to give your body time to process food between your eating windows.

Polls answered by people who have adopted this lifestyle indicate that most of them are happy with the results. Intermittent fasting is a very effective means of weight loss as it improves the metabolic rate of the body, as well as triggers cell autophagy. The good thing about intermittent fasting is that it allows you to partake of your favorite foods without making you feel guilty, which is a contrast to fad diets that insist on eating things like raw food and plant-based foods.

How to Practice Intermittent Fasting

There are a couple of ways to practice intermittent fasting. These are the three most popular ways:

- **The 16/8 method**

In this method, you are supposed to fast for 16 hours. Your eating window is restricted to eight hours every day. For instance, you might choose to only eat between twelve noon and eight in the evening.

- **Eat-Stop-Eat**

This fast involves irregular abstinence from food for a full 24 hours. You might decide to practice this once or twice every week. But when you fast, you must wait for 24 hours to pass before you indulge in the next meal. The eat-stop-eat method is very effective in not only weight loss but also in flushing out toxins from the body over the 24 hours you abstained from food.

- **The 5:2 Diet**

This type of intermittent fasting demands that you devote two days every week where you'll consume not more than 600 calories. Considering that the daily caloric requirement for the average person is 2000–2500, this type of fast will create a caloric deficit, and there's going to be weight loss as the body taps into its fat reservoirs for energy.

- **Alternate-Day Fasting**

This type of fasting requires that you skip one day and fast the next day. Depending on the intensity you want, you might choose to have a zero calorie intake or restrict your calorie intake to not more than 600. Alternate-day fasting is suitable for people who have experience with fasting and only want to escalate to amplify the benefits. A newbie should start with small fasts.

Pros and Cons of Intermittent Fasting

Intermittent fasting helps you save up on weekly food costs. That's a big advantage in these hard economic times. Food can be a very expensive affair especially if you eat out.

Intermittent fasting allows you to focus on your life goals. The energy that would have gone into looking for or preparing your next meal is used up to attain your important goals. Intermittent fasting has the potential to improve your emotional being and reduce anxiety—all of which make your life more stress-free.

Intermittent fasting is doable and safe. This means that it is free of complications and there's nothing to hold back anyone that wants to go into it. This is unlike other methods of weight loss like fad diets where some foods might be hard to access or expensive, or you dislike them.

Intermittent fasting improves the body's sensitivity to insulin, and by extension, it improves the metabolic rate of your body.

Moving on to the cons—the biggest disadvantage of intermittent fasting is the social dynamics. For instance, you might be out with friends when they decide to "pop in a joint" and then it's going to be strange to explain that you won't eat or maybe you'll defy your fasting routine and eat anyway, in which case you have cheated yourself.

Intermittent fasting doesn't seem to have a coherent and stable method. There are so many variations that dilute the philosophy of fasting. It almost feels like I can even come out with my style and popularize it. So, intermittent fasting lacks in originality.

Finding Your Ideal Intermittent Fasting Plan

The first and most important thing is to determine your health condition. If your body can permit you to indulge in intermittent fasting then, by all means, go ahead. If you are a beginner, you should start small, which means don't go from regular meals and start practicing 24-hour fasts. That's counterproductive. Make sure you have some experience before you fast for an extended period of time.

You'll find that what works for someone won't necessarily work for everybody else. So what's one supposed to do? Test, test, test. At one point you will find a variation of the intermittent fast that will fit perfectly into your life. It's all about finding what really works for you and then committing to the routine.

In my experience, I have found the 16:8 to be the best. This type of intermittent fast requires that you abstain from food for 16 hours and then indulge for 8 hours. For most followers of this routine, they like to have their eating window between 12:00 PM and 20:00 PM. The 16-hour fast will be inclusive of sleep, which makes it less severe.

This method is extremely efficient in weight loss, and most people have reported success. However, you must stick to the routine for a while before you can see any results. Don't do it for just one day and climb on the weighing machine only to find that there are no changes and then give up.

To improve the success of fasting intermittently, stick to a balanced diet during your eating windows, and don't take the fast as an excuse for indulging in unhealthy foods.

Step-By-Step Process of Fasting For a Week

The first step is to certify that you are in perfect condition. Get an appointment with your doctor and perform a whole health analysis to get a clean bill of health. Remember to always start with a small fast and gradually build up.

- **Day one**

When you wake up, forgo breakfast and opt for a glass of water or black coffee. Then go on about your work as you normally do. Around noon, your eating window opens. Now you are free to indulge in the food of your choice, but make sure that they are nutritious foods because unhealthy foods will water down your efforts. Your eating window should close at 20:00 PM, and from 20:01 pm to 12:00 pm the next day, don't consume anything else besides water.

- **Day two**

On day two, your body should have started to protest over the sudden calorie reduction, and so you'll be likely experiencing an irritable mood, lightheadedness, and a small headache. When you wake up, no matter how strong the urge to eat might be, just push it back, and the only thing you should consume is water or black coffee. At noon, your eating window opens, and you're free to eat until 8 pm.

- **Day three**

When you wake up, take a glass of water or black coffee. Chances are that your body has started to adjust to the reduced daily caloric intake. It has switched to burning fats. At twelve noon, when your eating window opens, consume less food than you did yesterday and the day before, so that the body has even lesser calories to work with. The body should adapt to this pretty swiftly.

- **Day four**

In the morning, take a glass of water or black coffee and go about your business. When your eating window opens, eat as much food as you ate yesterday, but in the evening, resist the urge to drink anything.

- **Day five**

When you wake up, take a glass of water or black coffee. During your eating window, eat less food than you did previously. At night, resist the urge to drink water.

- **Day six**

When you wake up, resist the urge to drink water or even coffee. In your eating window, choose not to eat at all, and at night give in to the temptation and drink water or black coffee.

- **Day seven**

When you wake up, take a glass of water or black coffee. In your eating window, resume eating, but only take a small portion, and just before you close the eating window, eat again, except it should be a slightly larger meal than previously. Before you sleep, take another glass of water or black coffee. Fast till your next eating window, and then you may resume your normal eating habits. At this point, you will have lost weight and experienced a host of other benefits attached to intermittent fasting.

Summary

Intermittent fasting features a cycle of fasting interrupted by an eating window. Some of the methods of intermittent fasting include the 16:8, eat-stop-eat, 5:2, and alternate-day fasting. The best approach to intermittent fasting is context-based in the sense that only you can know what works for you. The most popular form of intermittent fasting is the 16:8. In this method, you fast for 16 hours and then an eating window of 8 hours. The biggest advantage of intermittent fasting is that it announces relief to your pocket. The "food budget" goes into other uses. The amount of time that it takes to prepare meals is a real hassle, but intermittent fasting frees up your time so you can be more productive. The entry barrier is nonexistent too. This means anyone can practice intermittent fasting because there are no barriers or things to buy—a stark contrast to other weight loss methods like fad diets that may be both inconveniencing and expensive.

Chapter 7: Longer Periods of Fasting

What is Fasting for Longer Periods?

Fasting for longer periods is reserved for people who have a bit of experience with fasting. A newbie shouldn't get into it.

It is basically desisting from food for not less than 24 hours, but not more than, say, 48 hours. You may increase the success of the fast by making it a dry fast. In a dry fast, you won't have the luxury of drinking water or any other low-calorie drink like black coffee.

Fasting for longer periods requires that you prepare emotionally, mentally, and physically. The buildup to your fast is an especially important part. Your food consumption should be minimal.

Fasting for a longer period helps you achieve much more results because the body will be subjected to an increased level of strain.

However, you must take care to know when to stop. In some instances, the body might rebel by either catching an infection or shutting down critical functions, and in such times it is prudent to call off the fast.

During longer fasts, you should abstain from strenuous exercises, because the body will be in a state of energy conservation, and the available energy is purposed for physiological functions.

With the wrong approach, long fasts might become disastrous. That's why it is always important to seek clearance from your doctor first before you go into the fast. And to flush out toxins, ensure you have a steady intake of water.

It is estimated that weight loss in longer fasts averages around one to two pounds every day.

How to Fast for Longer Periods

The main reason that people go into longer fasts is to obviously lose weight. But you might want to fast to reach other purposes such as flushing toxins from your body or heightening your mental capabilities. Also, a longer fast is recommended if you are going into a surgery.

The response to a fast is different for everyone. If it is your first time, please take great care by getting medical clearance.

As your fast approaches, you might want to minimize your food consumption to get used to managing hunger.

Next, you should clear away items that might ruin your focus or tempt you to backslide. You might want to give your kitchen a total makeover by, for instance, clearing away the bad food. It is much easier to manage cravings when they are out of sight than when they are within easy reach.

Always start small. Before you deprive yourself food for over 24 hours, you should first get a taste of what food deprivation for 8 hours feels like, and if you can handle that, then you're ready to step up your game. While you fast, you should be very aware of the ranges of effects that your body experiences. You might feel dizzy, lightheaded, sleepy, or distressed, and these are okay reactions. Things that are not okay are infections and prolonged aches of body parts. If your body responds to fasting unfavorably, you should stop the fast.

Pros and Cons of Fasting for Longer Periods

If you have always been motivated to clear away the stubborn fat in your body, but have never found an efficient method, then the answer is to fast for a longer period.

When you go on a longer fast, the body uses up all glycogen in the first 24 hours, and then it switches to burning fats. A longer fast guarantees quick weight loss.

A longer fast saves you money. Food is an expensive affair, especially if you eat out. With a longer fast, it means you are staying away from food, and are thus saving on food costs.

Besides the benefit of optimizing your health, a longer fast will strengthen both your willpower and mental sharpness, which are two necessary factors in attaining success.

Fasting for a longer period helps you appreciate the taste of food. By the time you're done fasting, you'll want to indulge your appetite, and food will suddenly taste so sweet. The scarcity factor elevates the value of food.

A longer fast has cons, too. One of the biggest cons is the strain that it puts on your body. When your body goes from relying on glycogen into fats as a source of energy, nasty side effects are bound to come up—for instance, headaches, nausea, and lightheadedness.

Another con is that fasting for a longer period might open you up to disease. As much as fasting renews your immune system, your body still needs robust energy to function optimally. Fasting puts your body into a state of conserving energy which makes it easy for disease to attack.

Step-By-Step Process of Fasting for Longer Periods

When you decide to go on a fast for a longer period, you must realize that you are signing up for a real challenge. The body's immediate response to a fast is raising the hunger hormone to alert you to look for food. Now, fighting off that urge takes a lot of willpower. In some regard, it's why fasting might be considered a test of discipline because not so many people can withstand it.

So here's the step-by-step process of going on a fast for longer periods:

Preparation

The first major thing is to ensure that your body is in a condition that will allow you to fast, without any complications. In other words, consult your doctor for a checkup.

Reduce your food intake in the days leading up to your fast so that your body can get accustomed to staying without food. Once your body is familiar with the feeling of food deprivation, you are ready to move forward.

In the morning of your fast, drink lots of water. It is critical for flushing out toxins and reducing stomach acidity when your stomach secretes acids in anticipation of food. Your water intake should be regular and spread out through the day.

Rather than lying down and wearing a look of self-pity, just go on about your work as you normally would, provided it is not a very focus-oriented job like performing surgeries.

You should stay the whole day without food and then go to bed. On the following morning, your hunger pangs will be even more amplified, at which point you are to mitigate the hunger with a drink of water and then maintain the fast for another 24 hours. 48 hours are enough for a longer fast, and the weight loss should be dramatic. After the fast, don't immediately go back to eating heavy amounts of food, but rather ease your way into a lighter diet.

Chapter 8: Extended Fasting

How to Fast for Extended Periods

Fasting for an extended period is an extreme form of fasting that demands you abstain from food from anywhere between three days to seven days. If you can deny yourself food for more than three days, you should be proud of yourself, because not so many people have that kind of determination.

Fasting for an extended period of time amplifies the results of a longer fast. When you go for an extended period of time without food, you will allow yourself to experience a range of different feelings. At the initial stage there is distress, and towards the end your feelings become tranquil.

Considering that this is an especially long fast, you are supposed to take a very keen listen to the response by your body. If your body sends out the message that it is under massive strain, now it's time to stop the fast. Cases where it's appropriate to stop include developing stomach ulcers, throat infection, and loss of consciousness.

You should eat lighter meals as you approach the start of your fast. During the fast, your water intake should be regular. When you complete the fast, the transition to your normal eating life should be slow and gradual, starting with lighter meals.

Fasting for an extended period has the biggest potential of going wrong. The prolonged food deprivation in itself may do more good than harm. There is also the possibility of slightly altering your body's physiological functions. Still, the benefits of an extended fast outweigh the negatives.

Pros and Cons of Fasting for Extended Periods

The biggest advantage of fasting for an extended period of time is the discipline it instills in you. When you go for a prolonged period without eating food, your body will respond by increasing hunger pangs. It takes extreme willpower to keep going. This experience can help you build your self-control and discipline in real life.

An extended fast is very effective in banishing stubborn fat. Most people who are obese will tell you that they are trying to lose weight, but the fat is stubborn. Guess what, their methods are ineffective. However, if they had the will and courage to go on an extended fast, then they'd experience a rapid weight loss and reach their desired weight.

Extended fasting promotes a high rate of cell replenishing. When the body goes for days without food, it turns in on itself and begins to digest its cells—the weak and damaged cells—to provide nutrition for the healthy cells. The elimination of weak and damaged cells creates room for new and healthy ones.

The biggest disadvantage for an extended period of fasting is the risk of complications that you put your body into. Some complications might be instant whereas others may develop long after the fast. The biggest risk is catching an infection. If you're unlucky enough that you catch some disease in your fast, your immune system will be overwhelmed.

Another huge miss about extended fasting is the disconnect it encourages in your normal life. When you are fasting, you won't be able to share a meal with your friends or family, and that can be a big inconvenience. It can make people "talk."

Step-By-Step Process of Fasting for Extended Periods

When you get clearance from a medical professional, you should start by preparing for the extended fast. Ideally, if you are getting into an extended fast, you should have experience with either intermittent fasting, longer fasting or both. The more your body is familiar with food deprivation, the better the outcome.

On the start of your extended fast, you should consume only water or black coffee, and throughout the rest of the day, observe regular water consumption. It will aid in flushing out toxins and other harmful elements from your body.

During the fast, you should keep your normal work schedule, as opposed to being inactive, because inactivity will worsen your hunger pangs. The standard response to hunger pangs should be water consumption.

On the second day, first thing in the morning is to consume more water. This water is very critical in flushing out toxins and keeping your body cells hydrated as well as regulating autophagy. However, if you want to increase the success rate of the fast, you might consider eliminating water. One of the side effects of this type of fast is a dry mouth. A dry mouth has the potential of being very distressing. For purposes of safety, always hydrate yourself.

On the third day, wake up and consume water or black coffee. At this point, your body is subsisting on its fat reserves, and the weight loss is evident. Your body has potentially minimized hunger pangs to manageable levels. Keep yourself busy. Otherwise, inactivity will provoke hunger.

From the fourth day up until the seventh, keep the same routine. When you come to the end of your fast, realize that your body will be in starvation mode, so don't immediately consume large amounts of food. Instead, ease your way back into a normal eating schedule.

Chapter 9: The Eating Window

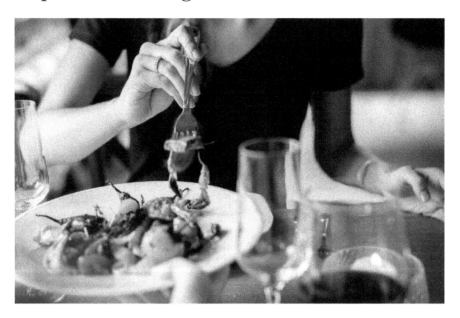

What is the Eating Window?

The eating window is the period of time that you are allowed to indulge in foods and one that precedes a period of fasting. The eating window comes around on a cycle, and you should adhere to it by only eating when the window opens and abstaining from food the rest of the time.

The hours are not set in stone. You are free to choose your eating window in a way that works for you. Most people who practice intermittent fasting seem to adhere to an eight-hour eating window followed by a sixteen-hour fast. Commonly, the eight-hour window opens at around 12:00 PM and goes all the way to 20:00 PM. During this time, you may indulge in your favorite foods. However, past 20:00 PM, you are supposed to observe the fast.

The 16:8 method of intermittent fasting appeals to many people because the 16 hours of fasting are inclusive of the bed-time. If you are not into waiting for sixteen hours before you partake of food, you may lessen the hours, so that you will have frequent eating windows between your fasts.

It is generally more fruitful to have a small eating window followed by a long period of fast.

It's also important to choose an eating window that optimizes your health. For instance, eating during the day is of much benefit than eating at night. This is because the body puts more calories to use during the day as opposed to while you are asleep. Also, adhere to a good diet, or else your gains will be neutralized by a bad diet.

What to Eat

The reason why intermittent fasting appeals to so many people is the nonexistent dietary rules common in alternative weight loss methods like fad diets. In intermittent fasting, you are free to eat the foods of your choice, and the main thing is to restrict your caloric intake.

You are free to consume the foods that delight you, but be careful not to fall in the pit of overcompensation. You are at risk of misleading yourself into consuming unhealthy foods during your eating window under the delusion that fasting will take care of it. Truth is, some of the fast foods we indulge are so calorie-laden that it would take a prolonged fast (not intermittent) to eliminate their fat from our bodies.

Limit your intake of red meat. As much as intermittent fasting is lenient when it comes to diet, it is widely known that red meat causes more harm than good. So, you might want to limit its intake or eliminate it altogether.

Fruits are a source of essential nutrients for the body. Always make sure to include fruits like bananas, avocados, and apples into your meals. Fruits help reduce inflammation and are critical in optimizing the physiological functions of the body.

Vegetables should be in your meals. People who claim that vegetables taste bad are just unimaginative cooks. Vegetables do taste good. And some of the health benefits of vegetable include strengthening your bones, stabilizing your blood sugar, boosting your brain health, and improving your digestive system.

Developing Discipline

It takes a lot of discipline to persevere through a fast. Think about it. The average person is accustomed to eating something every now and then. They cannot afford to hold back for even a couple more hours when lunch is due. The eating cycle never ends. And so a person who can decide to abstain from food and stick to their decision is a special kind of person— he/she is disciplined.

The biggest challenge when it comes to fasting for an extended period is to overcome the hunger pangs over the first few days. Your body floods you with the hunger hormone, pushing you to look for food. However, if you persevere through the first few days, your body will adjust to the food deprivation and switch to your stored fats as the alternative source of energy.

One of the things you must do to boost your self-control is to prepare your mind. When you have an idea of what to expect, the hunger will be more tolerable as opposed to if you're ignorant. Another thing to take into consideration is the weather. You don't want to fast during a cold season because fasting lowers your body temperature, and so you'll be hard-hit.

Another way of boosting your discipline is joining hands with people of the same goal. In this way, you can keep each other in check. When you are on a team or have a friend who practices fasting too, it will be easy to stick to your plan, as everybody will offer psycho-social support to everybody else. Sometimes, the difference between throwing in the towel and sticking to your guns is a kind word of encouragement.

Summary

The eating window is the period of time that you are allowed to indulge in foods and one that precedes a period of fasting. The eating window comes around on a cycle, and you should adhere to it by only eating when the window opens and abstaining from food the rest of the time. Intermittent fasting doesn't restrict the consumption of certain foods as is common for other weight loss methods such as fad diets. To boost the effectiveness of your fast, your diet should be balanced, which means it should include foods rich in minerals and vitamins. There also should be fruits and vegetables. Discipline is very important when it comes to fasting. It's what keeps you going when your body protests hunger. The most important step toward developing discipline is to first prepare mentally for the fast. Another way of developing discipline is by having a strong support system.

PART 2.3:

Targeted Fasting for Your Body Type

Chapter 10: Fasting For Weight Loss

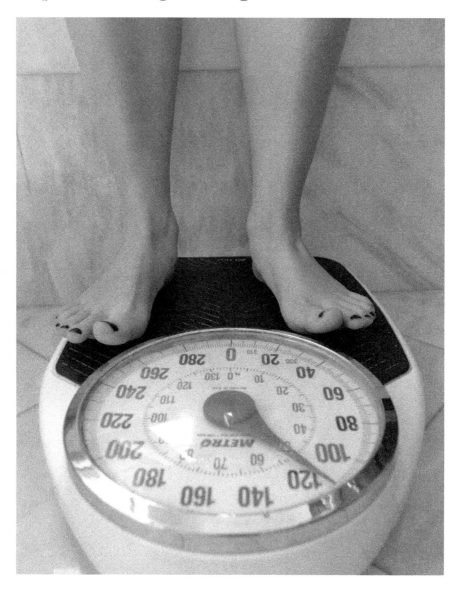

Why You'll Lose Weight through Fasting

Some of the methods of losing weight include fad diets, exercising, and supplements. However, these methods are not very effective, and in most cases, they cannot solve obesity on their own.

Fasting is easily the best method of not only reducing weight but also eliminating the stubborn lower-stomach fat. But why is it so?

First off, fasting optimizes the biological functions of your body. Fasting allows you to ease the load on your digestive system. The spare energy goes toward optimizing your physiological functions. For instance, improved digestion streamlines your bowel movement too. This efficacy in the physiological functions creates a compounding effect that leads to the shedding of dead weight, thus reducing an individual's weight and actually stabilizing it.

Another way in which fasting promotes weight loss is through cell autophagy. A dry fast is particularly what triggers cell autophagy. When the body uses up all its water, it now starts digesting the weak and damaged cells to provide water for the body cells that are in a much better state. Autophagy helps in eliminating dead and weak cells thereby making a person lighter.

Fasting plays a critical role in improving the metabolic health of an individual. With improved metabolism, the body can crunch more calories, and thus the individual's weight goes down.

Fasting improves insulin sensitivity. This helps the body to convert more sugars into energy. The body uses more calories, and as a result, there's a loss of weight.

In most obese people, the communication between their brain and ghrelin cells is warped, which makes them experience hunger all the time, even when they are full. Fasting helps remedy this problem, and obese people start receiving accurate signals when they are hungry.

Step-By-Step Process of Losing Weight through Fasting

- **Checkup**

First off, make sure that your body is in a condition that allows you to fast. Some of the people who are discouraged from the practice include pregnant women, nursing women, infants, sufferers of late-stage terminal illnesses, and those who are recovering from surgery.

- **Water**

Your body will respond to food deprivation by secreting acids and enzymes, and for that reason, always start your fast with consuming water. Regular water consumption will flush out the toxins and will also ease you from stomach pain.

- **Eating window**

Desist from food for at least 16 hours and then take a meal of your choice. The ideal eating window should be around eight hours. During this eight hour break, you are free to indulge. However, you must take care not to consume unhealthy foods. They will just neutralize your fasting efforts. Also, mind the portions. Simply because you have eight hours to feed doesn't mean you should fill up that period with food only.

- **Exercise**

Taking aerobic exercises, in particular, will have a dramatic effect on your weight loss. Aerobic exercises act like a calorie furnace. Also, exercises will increase the toxins in your body, and for that reason, keep yourself hydrated.

- **Breaking the fast**

At the end of your fast, never go right back into "heavy eating," but rather ease your way back by first consuming lighter foods. It'd be prudent of you to make fasting a part of your lifestyle. The key thing is to go with works for you. Most people seem to prefer intermittent fasting because it can fit in most people's lives. Prolonged fasting should be done sparingly as it carries the risk of developing complications.

Summary

Fasting has a positive impact on the rate of metabolism. When the metabolism rate is high, the energy output of the body goes up, and thus more calories are used up. This creates a caloric deficit and subsequent weight loss. Fasting promotes cell autophagy. Autophagy is the process where weak and damaged body cells are digested by the body. The elimination of weak body cells helps in weight reduction. High insulin resistance makes it hard for the body cells to absorb the sugars in the blood. But fasting reduces insulin resistance so that the body will use less insulin to convert sugars into energy. Before you go on a fast, you should get medical clearance. Some of the people who shouldn't get into a fast include the terminally ill, pregnant women, nursing women, and people who are recovering from surgery. It is important to take water throughout the fast to flush out toxins and mitigate the effect of stomach acids.

Chapter 11: Fasting for Type 2 Diabetes

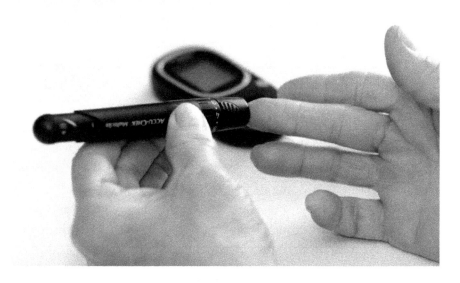

What is Type 2 Diabetes?

Type 2 diabetes is a disease that damages the ability of the pancreas to produce sufficient insulin. Insulin is the hormone produced by the pancreas, and its main function is to regulate the conversion of glucose into energy. The body cells of people who have type 2 diabetes are insensitive to insulin, and as such, they experience difficulty in converting sugars into energy. This condition is known as insulin resistance. It is characterized by the production of higher amounts of insulin, but the body cannot absorb it.

As to the origin of type 2 diabetes, scientists have established that it is genetic. The disease is handed down to progeny. Another leading cause of type 2 diabetes is obesity. Overweight people are much more likely to develop insulin resistance. There's a link between childhood obesity and development of type 2 diabetes in adulthood.

Another contributing factor is a metabolic syndrome. High insulin resistance is a result of increased blood pressure and cholesterol. Excessive sugars produced by the liver may also be a trigger.

The symptoms of type 2 diabetes cover a wide range. They include thirst, frequent peeing, hazy vision, irritability, tiredness, and yeast infections.

The risk of developing type 2 diabetes can be greatly minimized by taking the following actions:

Losing weight. Weight loss improves insulin sensitivity, and thus the buildup of insulin in the blood is eliminated. Also, there's more conversion of sugars into energy.

Balanced diet. You should consume foods that are sources of minerals and vitamins. Increase your intake of fruits and vegetables. Minimize your consumption of sugars and red meat.

The Role of Insulin in the Body

The insulin hormone is produced by the pancreas. Its key role is to regulate blood sugar. Increased insulin resistance might lead to type 2 diabetes. Insulin plays the critical role of facilitating absorption of sugars into body cells. In this way, insulin helps to reduce the blood sugar level. Another important role of insulin is to modify the activity of enzymes. The enzymes are secreted by the body when there's food in the stomach. Insulin regulates the activity of enzymes.

Insulin helps the body recover quickly. When your body is recovering from an injury or illness, insulin plays a critical role in speeding up the healing process by transporting amino acids to cells.

Insulin promotes gut flora and thus improves gut health. This improves bowel movement. Insulin also improves the excretion of harmful substances like sodium.

Insulin promotes brain health. It improves brain clarity by providing the essential nutrients to the brain.

Insulin plays a key role in determining the metabolism rate of the body. In instances of high insulin sensitivity, the blood glucose is easily absorbed into the cells, making for a high metabolic rate. But in instances of low insulin sensitivity, the process of converting sugars into energy becomes hard, and, consequently, there is a low metabolic rate.

Insulin is very important in the optimal functioning of your body. Some of the factors that improve the production of the insulin hormone are having a balanced diet, improving your brain health, having quality sleep, exercising, and staying in a pollution-free environment.

How Diabetes Affects both Production and Usage of Insulin

Diabetes is a major lifestyle disease all over the world. A person who has diabetes either cannot produce sufficient insulin, or their body cells are insensitive to insulin. Diabetes is broadly classified into two types: type 1 and type 2.

People who suffer from type 1 diabetes produce little to no insulin. This slows down the rate of conversion of sugars into energy. A low level of insulin is mainly a result of the immune system attacking the pancreas and curtailing its ability to produce sufficient insulin. Also, low insulin levels might be a result of weakened and damaged body cells. Type 1 diabetes commonly affects young people. One of the corrective measures is to administer insulin through injections.

Symptoms of type 1 diabetes include dehydration, constant urge to urinate, hunger (even after eating), unexplained weight loss, blurry vision, exhaustion, and bad moods.

Type 2 diabetes is the most common form of diabetes. People who suffer from type 2 diabetes have a high insulin resistance. Their body cells are averse to insulin. Types 2 diabetes is treated by increasing insulin sensitivity.

Symptoms of type 2 diabetes include tiredness, never-ending thirst, constant urge to pee, irritability, weak immune, and shivering.

The pancreas is the organ that produces insulin. When we consume food, blood sugar rises. The pancreas releases insulin to facilitate the conversion of sugars into energy. But someone who suffers from diabetes either lacks sufficient insulin or their body cannot use the released insulin. This results in increased blood sugar levels. This scenario presents risks such as the development of heart disease and stroke.

How Blood Sugar Responds To Fasting

A carbohydrate metabolism test is crucial in determining how blood sugar responds to fasting. The test is conducted on diabetics. During a fast, the levels of plasma glucose go up. People with diabetes either cannot produce sufficient insulin, or their bodies are resistant to insulin. Non-diabetics, though, produce insulin that brings down the levels of glucose through absorption.

Diet greatly affects the blood sugar rate-of-increase. For instance, a big serving of food will trigger a high level of blood sugar, and sugar-laden foods like cake, bread, and fries will also increase the blood sugar level.

People with type 1 diabetes lack sufficient insulin because their immune system attacks the pancreas, while people with type 2 diabetes are insensitive to insulin. So in both cases, there is a high level of blood sugar.

The levels of blood glucose during fasting give us insight into how the cells respond to blood sugar. A high level of blood glucose is indicative of the body's ability to lower blood glucose, and the conclusion might be either high insulin resistance or insufficient insulin production. Prolonged fasting has the effect of minimizing blood glucose levels. The sugars in the blood get used up, albeit slowly.

There are two methods of testing the level of blood sugar: the traditional blood sugar test, and the glycosylated hemoglobin (HbAlc). The glycosylated hemoglobin test is for checking how blood glucose has been changing. The traditional method of checking blood sugar involves daily tests which may be conducted by the affected person.

Developing Your Fasting Regimen

There are some fasting regimens. All of them have their pros and cons. They are only as good as the person trying to follow them. During fasts, it is recommended to take water to flush out toxins and also to mitigate hunger. However, if you want to improve the success rate of your fast, you might consider dry fasts, where you don't consume any fluid.

You may perform a fast for as short a time as a couple of hours or as long as a full week (and maybe even more, depending on your stamina). However, if your goal is to lose weight, then shorter fasts are more effective. For instance, intermittent fasting is many times more fruitful than prolonged fasting, but ultimately, you get to choose what you feel will work for you.

Short fasts allow you to go through a cycle of fasting and eating windows. You start by creating a plan in which you detail your period of fasting and when your eating window opens. During the eating window, it is advisable to consume unprocessed foods and avoid sugar-laden foods. This will boost your insulin sensitivity.

Long fasts have their benefits too, but on the whole, they are much less rewarding than short fasts. The strain associated with long fasts make you susceptible to infections and might, in the worst case scenario, rewire your physiological functions.

Things to Incorporate to Make Fasting Safe for Diabetics

When a diabetic goes on a fast, their body secretes the glucagon hormone, which leads to a spike in the blood sugar level. Thus, a diabetic should start by informing themselves properly before they deprive themselves of food.

The first thing is to determine whether they are fit to fast. A diabetic person should seek medical clearance before they attempt fasting. A person with advanced diabetes will have a low blood sugar level. If they go on a fast, they risk falling into a coma. A medical professional offers the best counsel as to how to conduct the fast and for how long.

For type 1 diabetics, it is important to have a test kit to observe the fluctuation of blood sugar throughout the fast. This helps in tweaking the fast or deciding whether to call it off.

Another safety measure is to have a confidant know of their fasting. The psycho-social support offered by a confidant would keep them going. The confidant should be someone in their close proximity that can monitor their progress.

Diabetics should indulge in a balanced diet during their eating window. A balanced diet comprises of foods rich in minerals and vitamins. One common thing that fasting induces is cravings. Fast foods, for instance, are sugar-laden and they have no real nutritional value. Indulging in fast foods during eating windows only negates the effectiveness of the fast.

A diabetic should know when to quit and how to quit. If there is a massive fluctuation of blood glucose, or if a complication develops, then that's a hint to quit. Towards the end of the fast, a diabetic should consume light meals first, and then transition back to their normal eating patterns.

Role of Supplements

A supplement is a substance that enhances the food that a person eats. The common types of ingredients in supplements include vitamins, minerals, botanicals, amino acids, enzymes, organ tissues, and glandulars. The supplements are critical in optimizing nutritional value of food. The water-soluble ingredients of supplements are metabolized and eliminated from the body same day, while fat-soluble elements may be stored in the body for several days or even weeks. Supplements may be taken on either a daily basis or alternately—depending on the elements they provide to the body. One should always seek the guidance of a medical professional about the number of supplements to consume.

Supplements are not as critical during short fasts as they are in prolonged fasts. The body is a store of many nutritional elements, and fasting induces the body to tap into its reservoirs, but it is still important to take supplements to discourage nutrition deficiency. Fat-soluble vitamins need to be taken alongside fats to make for easy absorption. They include vitamin A, vitamin D, vitamin E, and vitamin K. They are kept in body cells too. Water-soluble vitamins are eliminated on the same day, especially if your body is well hydrated. Water-soluble vitamins include B3, B2, B1, and acids. If you have a poor diet, water-soluble vitamins are stable sources of nutrition.

The primary function of supplements is to improve the nutritional value of a person's diet by supplying vital elements that are not easily accessible. Taking supplements while on a fast helps mitigate the side effects of fasting such as headaches and cramps.

Types of Supplements that Stabilize Electrolytes

Sodium. The intake of Sodium is dependent upon your level of physical activity. Generally, if you engage in tougher physical exercises, you should take a high dose. Sodium is vital in eliminating cramps and various pains in the body.

Potassium. This supplement is vital for the optimal functioning of the heart. Potassium deficiency is normally accompanied by problems such as increased heartbeat and blood pressure. Potassium also helps in the flow of blood. A person with potassium deficiency is bound to experience exhaustion and constant lethargic feeling.

Magnesium. People who are lacking in this vital nutrient experience a range of problems like low energy, anxiety, insomnia, indigestion, muscle aches, poor heart health, and migraines. Magnesium supplements help your body absorb magnesium at a higher rate. Magnesium should be taken alongside food as opposed to plainly for maximum health benefit.

Zinc. This supplement is very crucial in improving the health of an individual. It regulates appetite, improves taste, promotes weight loss, minimizes hair loss, mitigates digestive problems, and cures chronic fatigue. Additionally, zinc improves nerve health and boosts testosterone.

Zinc, too, should be consumed alongside other meals for maximum health benefits.

Calcium. This supplement helps in strengthening the musculoskeletal frame of an individual, heart health, and reduces the risk of developing ailments like cancer and diabetes. Calcium and magnesium should be taken at separate times to avoid stunted absorption rates.

Iodine. Iodine is crucial in improving thyroid health. The thyroid gland secretes hormones that play a vital role in the basal metabolic rate.

How to Keep Insulin Levels Low

This hormone produced by the pancreas facilitates the absorption of sugars into body cells. The insulin levels should be stable for optimum metabolism to take place. High levels of insulin might lead to serious complications like high blood pressure. Someone with a high blood glucose level needs to lower their blood sugar level, else they may suffer serious health complications. Here are some of the ways to keep insulin levels low.

Diet. Your diet will have a direct impact on your blood sugar levels. Sugary, fat-laden foods will raise your blood glucose through the roof. On the other hand, a low-carb diet will help keep your blood glucose levels down.

Portion. There is a direct correlation between the portion of your food and your blood sugar levels. A giant portion of your favorite dish will lead to a surge in blood glucose. On the other hand, a small portion will keep your blood sugar stable. Bearing this in mind, you should aim to take small portions of food, as they minimize the fluctuation of blood glucose levels.

Exercise regularly. You can bring the high blood sugar levels down through exercise. When you exercise, your body powers your activities with the glucose in your blood. So exercises—and in particular, aerobics—can lead to low blood glucose levels.

Drink water constantly. Staying hydrated is also important in keeping the blood sugar level down. Water will flush out toxins and help streamline your metabolism.

Avoid alcohol. Alcohol not only lowers your inhibitions and makes you indulge in unhealthy foods like fries and roast meat, but it is also calorie-packed. If you aim to minimize your blood sugar, restrict your alcohol intake or drop it altogether.

What Causes Insulin Resistance?

Insulin is produced by the pancreas, and its work is to facilitate absorption of glucose into body cells. Insulin resistance is a condition where body cells are insensitive to insulin. For that reason, the rate of conversion of sugars into energy is affected. What are some of the causes of this condition?

Obesity. Most obese people have a ton of toxic elements stashed in their body. The combination of high blood sugar levels and toxic elements promote cellular inflammation. These cells naturally become insulin resistant.

Inactivity. Insulin resistance is common in people who hardly ever move their limbs. They don't perform any physical activity, so their energy requirement (output) is minimal. This creates some sort of "cell apathy" and promotes insulin resistance.

Sleep apnea. This is a sleep disorder characterized by faulty breathing. People who suffer from sleep apnea snore loudly and also feel tired after a night's sleep. Studies have shown a link between sleep apnea and development of insulin resistance in body cells.

High blood pressure. High blood pressure or hypertension is a degenerative medical issue where the blood pressure in blood vessels is more than 140/90 mmHg. Hypertension makes the heart's task of pumping out blood more difficult and may contribute to complications such as atherosclerosis, stroke, and kidney disease. Studies have shown a correlation between people with high blood pressure and the development of insulin resistance.

Smoking. The habit of smoking can give you many health complications. One of them is the risk of cancer development. Additionally, smoking seems to promote insulin resistance.

How Insulin Resistance Affects the Body

Insulin resistance makes it hard for the body cells to absorb sugars, which leads to high blood glucose levels. Some of the causes of insulin resistance include obesity, poor diet, sleep disorders, and sedentary lifestyle.

The American Diabetes Association (ADA) has stated that there is a 70% chance for people with insulin resistance to develop type 2 diabetes if they don't change their habits.

Insulin resistance may trigger the development of acanthosis nigricans, a skin condition in which dark spots cover parts of the body, especially the neck region.

Insulin resistance enhances weight gain, because it slows down base metabolism, causing a surge of blood sugar levels. Insulin carries off the excess blood sugar into fat stores, and thus, the person gains weight.

Insulin resistance promotes high blood pressure. The elevated blood glucose levels cause the heart to have to struggle with pumping more blood, causing high blood pressure.

Insulin resistance causes constant thirst and hunger pangs. Insulin resistance promotes the miscommunication between brain receptors and body cells. Thus, the brain activates the hunger hormone and makes the person eternally hungry. If not corrected, this leads to overeating and eventually chronic obesity.

Insulin resistance weakens the body. Insulin resistance leads to low energy output. And for that reason, the body doesn't have a lot of energy to use up, which makes the person feel (and look) weak.

Insulin resistance makes you urinate frequently; the condition affects the efficiency of physiological functions, and one of the results is a constant need to urinate.

Insulin resistance makes the body more susceptible to attack by diseases.

The Role of Amylin

Amylin is a protein hormone. It is produced by the pancreas alongside insulin. Amylin helps in glycemic control by promoting the slow emptying of the gastric and giving feelings of satisfaction. Amylin discourages the upsurge of blood glucose levels.

Amylin is part of the endocrine system, and it plays a critical role in glycemic control. The hormone is secreted by the pancreas, and its main function is to slow down the rate of appearance of nutritional elements in the plasma. It complements insulin.

Amylin and Insulin are secreted in a ratio of 1:100. Amylin delays gastric emptying and decreases the concentration of glucose in the plasma, whereas insulin facilitates absorption of sugars into cells. Diabetic people lack this hormone.

The amylin hormone can coalesce and create amyloid fibers, which may help in destroying diabetes. Amylin is secreted when there is the stimulus of nutrition in the blood. Unlike insulin, it is not purged in the liver but by renal metabolism.

Recent studies have shown the effect of amylin on the metabolism of glucose. In rats, amylin promoted insulin resistance.

Amylin slows down the food movement through the gut. As the food stays longer in the stomach, the rate of conversion of these foods to sugars will be slower.

Amylin also prevents the secretion of glucagon. Glucagon causes a surge in blood sugar level. Amylin prevents the inappropriate secretion of glucagon, which might cause a post-meal spike in blood sugar.

Amylin enhances the feeling of satiety. By reducing appetite, amylin ensures low blood glucose levels.

How Amylin Deficiency Affects Your Body

Amylin regulates the concentration of glucose in the blood by preventing the secretion of glucagon and slowing down the movement of food along the gut. People who suffer from diabetes have an amylin deficiency that causes excessive amounts of glucose to flow into the blood.

Increased insulin. A deficiency in amylin causes an extreme surge in blood glucose levels. To mitigate this spike, the pancreas secretes more insulin to help in the absorption of sugars into body cells. Increased levels of insulin in the blood might lead to complications.

Insulin resistance. Amylin deficiency eventually leads to high blood glucose levels. This might cause insulin resistance in body cells and, in worst case scenarios, it might trigger the immune system to attack the pancreas. High insulin levels in the blood might trigger memory loss and might even induce a coma.

Diabetes. Amylin deficiency leads to the overproduction of insulin, which, in the long run, impairs the pancreas. When the normal working of the pancreas is damaged, diabetes may develop.

Weight gain. Amylin deficiency promotes insulin resistance. When body cells become insensitive to insulin, there is less sugar converted into energy. So, the blood glucose level remains high. Insulin is responsible for carrying off these sugars to be stored as fats. Instead of these sugars being used as energy, they end up being stored as fat in the cells, which is the start of weight gain.

Headache. Thanks to insulin resistance, the body cells lack a reliable source of energy, which causes the body to switch to burning fats as an alternative energy source. One of the side effects of this process is normally headache and nausea.

The Insulin Resistance Diet

Insulin resistance causes slower absorption of sugars into body cells. This condition is rampant in obese people and diabetics. It is projected that the number of diabetics in the next 20 years will be over 320 million. This indicates a very worrying trend of diabetes. One of the things we can do to fight against diabetes is to improve our diet. Studies have shown that weight loss is a very effective means of minimizing insulin resistance. Here are the components of an insulin resistant diet:

Low carbs. Food high in carbs are responsible for blood sugar spikes. High levels of blood glucose promote insulin resistance. To ensure a stable blood glucose level, you should stick to low-carb foods.

Avoid sugary drinks. The American Diabetes Association advises against consumption of sugary drinks. These drinks with high sugar content include fruit juice, corn syrup, and other concentrates. Sugary drinks have a high sugar content, and they spike blood sugar levels. So, it'd be prudent to stay away from sugary drinks.

More fiber. Fiber is important in reducing the blood glucose levels. It improves the digestive health and improves blood circulation.

Healthy fats. Monounsaturated fats are very critical in improving heart health and regulating insulin levels.

Protein. Studies show that dietary protein is beneficial for people who suffer from diabetes. Regular consumption of protein is important for muscle growth and bone mass.

Size. Instead of taking large servings of a meal, opt for smaller portions of food, so that your post-meal blood glucose levels may be stable.

The Best Food for Diabetics

Diabetics don't have the luxury of eating any food they might want. For instance, sugar-laden foods and high-fat foods would spike their blood sugar levels and worsen the condition. They should instead stick to foods that are sources of minerals and vitamins. Foods like:

Fish. Fish is an important source of omega-3 fatty acids. These fatty acids are especially great for people with heart health complications and those who are at risk of stroke. Omega three fatty acids also protect your blood vessels, as well as reduce inflammation. Studies show that people who consume fish on the regular have better heart health than those who don't.

Greens. They are very nutritious and have low calories. Leafy greens like kale and spinach are excellent sources of minerals and vitamins. Leafy greens reduce inflammation markers, as well improve blood pressure. They are also high in antioxidants.

Eggs. The good old egg has been abused at the hands of intellectual conmen who have long said, albeit incorrectly, that eggs are bad. Eggs are excellent for reducing heart disease complications and also decreasing inflammation markers. Regular consumption of eggs improves cholesterol and blood glucose levels.

Chia seeds. They are high in fiber, and this fiber is critical in lowering blood glucose levels as well as in slowing down the rate of movement of food along the gut.

Nuts. Nuts are both tasty and healthy. They are great sources of fiber and are low in carbs. Regular consumption improves heart health and reduces inflammation and improves blood circulation.

Summary

Type 2 diabetes is a degenerative disease that impairs the ability of the pancreas to produce insulin. The hormone insulin is produced by the pancreas, and its main function is to regulate the conversion of glucose to energy. The risk of developing diabetes can be greatly minimized by taking the two steps: losing weight and having a balanced diet. The number of people with diabetes is at an all-time high, and people in both developed and poor countries are battling the disease. Symptoms of type 2 diabetes include tiredness, never-ending thirst, the constant urge to pee, irritability, weak immune system, and shivering. A carbohydrate metabolism test determines how blood sugar reacts to fasting. During a fast, blood sugar levels go up. Supplements are necessary for supplying important nutrients that may not be in the diet. The intake of supplements should be daily for optimum results. The important supplements include sodium, potassium, magnesium, zinc, calcium, and iodine. These are some of the measures to take to keep insulin levels low: have a strict diet, consume small portions, exercise regularly, and drink water constantly.

Chapter 12: Fasting For Heart Health

How Fasting Improves Your Heart's Health

Numerous studies have shown that fasting has a positive impact on heart health. Many people who have gone on a fast have reported feeling energetic and livelier afterward, which could be attributed to improved blood flow and general heart health. However, you need to fast consistently to achieve results.

Improves your heartbeat. When you go on a fast, your body is free from the digestion load, and so it channels that energy into optimizing your physiological functions. Your heart stands to gain from the optimized body functions, especially improving your heartbeat.

Improves blood pressure. Studies show that fasting has a positive impact on blood pressure. The rate of blood pressure is affected by factors like weight gain and obesity. But since fasting helps in weight loss, it has the extended advantage of lowering blood pressure, which improves the overall heart health.

Reduces cholesterol. Regularly fasting helps in lowering bad cholesterol. Also, controlled fasting increases the base metabolic rate.

Improved blood vessel health. Fasting is critical in improving the health of blood vessels. When blood vessels are subjected to high blood pressure, they slowly start to wear out, and might eventually burst up—which could be fatal, especially in the case of arteries. But fasting helps reduce blood pressure and bad cholesterol. The result is improved blood flow and overall heart health.

Autophagy. Regular dry fasts trigger the body to digest its weak and damaged cells in a process known as autophagy. Cell autophagy is very crucial because it helps eliminate old and damaged cells and creates room for new cells. With a new batch of cells to work with, the heart health is given a tremendous boost.

Summary

Fasting has been shown to improve the health of the heart. When you are fasting, your body reserves energy that would have gone into digestion for purposes of improving the heart health. It can execute its physiological functions much better. Fasting has also been shown to improve blood pressure. Fasting helps reduce obesity and reduces weight gain. This causes massive improvement in blood pressure. Fasting also plays a critical role in reducing cholesterol. Bad cholesterol increases the rate of developing heart disease. Also, controlled fasting increases the base metabolic rate. Fasting also improves the health of blood vessels. High blood pressure might cause blood vessels to wear out slowly, but fasting has a restorative effect on the blood vessels. Fasting also allows the body to digest its weak cells and make room for new and powerful body cells.

Chapter 13: The General Results of Fasting

Positive Effects of Fasting

You will get varied results depending on your preferred method of fasting, whether it's intermittent fasting, alternate-day, or prolonged fasting. These are some of the positive effects of fasting:

Weight loss. Fasting is an efficient way of losing weight. A study in 2015 showed that alternate fasting for a week resulted in weight loss of up to seven percent. When your body uses up the glucose in your blood, it now turns to the fat reserves to power its bodily functions. This helps in achieving weight loss.

Release of the human growth hormone. The human growth hormone promotes the growth of muscles and reduces obesity. Fasting triggers the secretion of the human growth hormone. This hormone is very crucial in building your body cells.

Improves insulin sensitivity. Low insulin sensitivity restricts the absorption of sugars into body cells. This might lead to complications such as chronic weight gain. Fasting leads to high insulin sensitivity that helps in absorption of sugars into body cells.

Normalizes ghrelin levels. Ghrelin is the hunger hormone which sends out hunger signals. Most obese people have abnormal ghrelin hormone levels that keep them in a perpetual state of hunger. Fasting, however, remedies this situation by normalizing ghrelin hormone levels, and thus you can receive accurate signals about hunger.

Lowers triglyceride levels. Depriving yourself of food for a set period of time has the effect of lowering bad cholesterol, and in the process, triglycerides are reduced.

Slows down aging. Many studies have shown the link between fasting and increased longevity in animals. Fasting allows the body to cleanse itself, promotes cell autophagy, and in the long run, lengthens lifespan.

Negative Effects of Fasting

As much as fasting is a practice with many benefits, admittedly there is a dark side too. These are some of the negative effects of fasting:

Strained body. A prolonged fast might put a big deal of a strain on your body. This may alter—albeit slightly—the normal processes of your body. A prolonged fast might slow down the effectiveness of your body as the body adapts to survive on too little energy.

Headaches. Headaches are common during fasts, especially at the start. The headache is normally a response of the brain to diminished blood glucose levels that force the body to switch to burning fats as a source of energy.

Low blood pressure. Fasting is a major cause of low blood pressure. Low blood pressure slows down the conversion of sugars into energy. This may lead to complications such as temporary blindness and, in extreme cases, can induce a coma.

Eating disorders. For someone who's too eager, it is easy to abuse fasting and turn it into an eating disorder. The main aim of fasting is to improve health, but starving yourself and having an eating disorder is anything but healthy. Some of the eating disorders that people who fast are at risk of developing include anorexia and bulimia.

Cravings. The hunger triggered by fasting might cause us to overcompensate. We may develop cravings for fast foods and other unhealthy foods. During our eating window, we may find ourselves consuming a lot of unhealthy foods, under the delusion that the fast will override that.

Summary

Weight loss is one of the main benefits of fasting. When you fast, your blood glucose is diminished, and this forces your body to turn to fats as an alternative source of energy. Fasting also promotes the production of the human growth hormone. This is the hormone responsible for muscle growth. Fasting also improves insulin sensitivity. Low insulin sensitivity impairs the body's ability to convert sugars into energy. Fasting also leads to high insulin sensitivity that helps in the absorption of sugars into body cells. Fasting also helps normalize ghrelin levels. The ghrelin hormone is known as the hunger hormone. Most obese people have abnormally high ghrelin levels that give incorrect hunger signals and make the obese person perpetually hungry. Fasting helps in correcting this problem, and the obese person starts to receive accurate signals. The negative effects of fasting include straining the body, headaches, low blood pressure, and eating disorders.

PART 2.4:

Important Factors that Improve the Quality of Fasting

Chapter 14: Nutrition

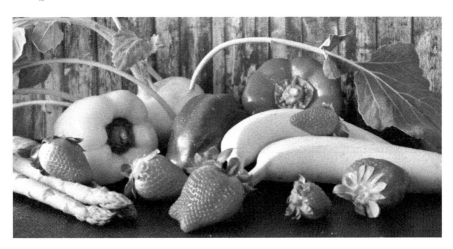

What Constitutes Good Nutrition?

Good nutrition implies a diet that contains all the required and important nutrients in appropriate proportions. When you fail to observe good nutrition, you risk developing complications from certain nutrient deficiencies. A good nutrition shouldn't be a one-off thing, but it should be a part of your lifestyle.

A great nutrition minimizes the risk of developing health complications such as diabetes, heart disease, and chronic weight gain. Here are the most important constituents of great nutrition:

- **Protein**

This nutrient is very important for muscle health, skin health, and hair. Also, it assists in the bodily reactions. Amino acids are essential for human growth and protein is stacked with amino acids. The best sources of protein include fish, eggs, and lentils.

- **Carbohydrates**

Carbohydrates are the main sources of energy for the body. They provide sugars that are converted into energy. There are two classes of carbohydrates: simple and complex. Simple carbohydrates are digested easily, and complex carbohydrates take time. Fruits and grains are some of the main sources of simple carbohydrates whereas beans and vegetables are sources of complex carbohydrates. For proper digestion, dietary fiber (carbohydrate) is needed. Men need a daily intake of 30 grams of fiber and women need 24 grams. Important sources of dietary fiber include legumes and whole grains.

- **Fats**

Fats play an essential role in health improvement. Both monounsaturated and polyunsaturated fats are healthy. Sources of monounsaturated fats include avocados and nuts. As for polyunsaturated fats, seafood is a major source. Unhealthy fats include trans fats and saturated fats, mostly found in junk food.

- **Vitamins**

Vitamins A, B, C, D, E, and K are necessary for the body's optimal functioning. A deficiency in the important vitamins can lead to serious health complications and weakened immune system.

- **Minerals**

Calcium, iron, zinc, and iodine are some of the essential minerals. They are found in a variety of foods including vegetables, grains, and meats.

- **Water**

Most of the human body is composed of water. It is a very essential nutrient for the proper functioning of the body.

Why Good Nutrition Is Important

The main reason why people ensure that they have a good nutrition is to improve their health. A good nutrition is essentially about consuming foods that are rich in vitamins, minerals, and fats. So, here are some of the reasons why good nutrition is vital.

Reduces risk of cancer. Good nutrition plays a vital role in optimizing your health. If you consume healthy food, you drastically reduce your chances of getting cancer, as many cancers are a result of bad lifestyle choices.

Reduces risk of developing high blood pressure. High blood pressure causes a strain on the heart. It also leads to the wearing and tearing of the blood vessels. Having good nutrition normalizes your blood pressure and thus improves your heart health.

Lowers cholesterol. Bad cholesterol leads to serious complications like heart disease. When you observe good nutrition that involves fruits and essential vitamins, the bad cholesterol is eliminated, thus improving the functioning of your body.

Increased energy. Bad food choices have a draining effect. However, nutritious foods replenish the body cells with vital nutrients, and thus the body is active. A nutritious diet is a key to improving productivity.

Improved immunity. Diseases are always looking for new victims. People who have a poor diet are bound to have a weak immune system. The weak immune system won't sufficiently protect them against attacks. On the other hand, people who consume a nutritious diet tend to have a strong immune system. This improved immunity keeps diseases at bay.

The Advantages of a High-Fat Diet

Many studies have shown that a low-carb, high-fat diet has many health benefits, including weight management, and reduced risk of diabetes, cancer, and Alzheimer's. A high-fat diet is characterized by low carbohydrate intake and high intake of fat. The low carbohydrate intake puts the body into ketosis, a condition that optimizes burning of fat and helps convert fat into ketone bodies that act as an energy source of the brain. These are some of the advantages of a high-fat diet:

Stronger immune system. Saturated fats are an ally of the immune system. They help fight off microbes, viruses, and fungi. Fats help in the fight against diseases. A great source of saturated fats includes butter and coconut.

Improves skin health and eyesight. When someone is lacking in fatty acids, they are likely to develop dry skin and eyes. Fatty acids help in improving skin elasticity and strengthening eyesight.

Lowers risk of heart disease. Saturated fats trigger production of good cholesterol, which is key in reducing the risk of heart disease. Saturated fats also help fight inflammation. A good source of saturated fats includes eggs and coconut oil.

Strong bones. Healthy fats improve the density of bones and thus minimize the risk of bone diseases. Fats promote healthy calcium metabolism. Fatty acids, too, play a critical role in minimizing the risk of bone complications such as osteoporosis.

Improves reproductive health. Fats play a critical role in the production of hormones that improve fertility in both men and women. A high-fat diet improves reproductive health and, in particular, the production of testosterone and estrogen.

Weight loss. A high-fat diet promotes high metabolism and, as a result, the body can crunch more calories, leading to weight loss.

Improved muscle gain. A high-fat diet promotes muscle gain. This is achieved through hormone production and speeding up cell recovery after strenuous exercise.

Role of Ketone Bodies

The three ketone bodies produced by the liver include acetoacetate, beta-hydroxybutyrate, and acetone. Ketone bodies are water-soluble, and it takes a blood or urine test to determine their levels.

Ketone bodies are oxidized in the mitochondria to provide energy. The heart uses fatty acids as fuel in normal circumstances, but during ketogenesis, it switches to ketone bodies. When the blood glucose levels are high, the body stores the excesses as fat. When you go for an extended period of time without eating, the blood glucose levels diminish. This triggers the body to convert fat into usable energy. Most body cells can utilize fatty acids, except the brain. The liver thus converts fats into ketone bodies and releases them into the blood to supply energy to the brain. When ketone bodies start to build up in the blood, problems might arise. An increase in the levels of acetone can induce acidosis, a condition where blood pH is lowered. Acidosis has a negative impact on most of the body cells, and in worst cases, it leads to death. With that in mind, it is prudent to replenish your body with carbohydrates as soon as ketosis kicks off. A person with type 1 diabetes is more susceptible to high levels of ketone bodies. For instance, when they fail to take an insulin shot, they will experience hypoglycemia. The combination of low blood glucose level and high glucagon level will cause the liver to produce ketone bodies at an alarming rate which might cause complications.

Benefits of the Ketogenic Diet

Here are some of the benefits associated with ketone bodies:

Treating Alzheimer's. Alzheimer's behaves in a way similar to diabetes. Essentially, it is the brain resisting insulin. Due to insulin resistance, the brain only gets minimal energy, which might cause the death of brain cells. However, ketone bodies are an alternative source of energy that the brain can utilize. Ketone bodies have been shown to prevent a buildup of compounds that enhance the development of Alzheimer.

Normalizes insulin production. Ketone bodies are only produced when blood glucose is low. For this reason, the pancreas stops pumping more insulin to aid in the absorption of sugars because the body has already switched into ketogenesis.

Regulates metabolism. Ketone bodies regulate metabolism through their effects on mitochondria. The mitochondria are the cells' power plants, and they respond better to energy from fats rather than glucose. In this sense, ketone bodies improve the functioning of the mitochondria.

Lowers hunger. When the body is utilizing ketone bodies, it seems that there's less of an urge to consume food. Ketogenesis regulates the hunger hormone. When a person is consuming fast foods, there is no end to the urge to take another serving. Eventually, this leads to weight gain.

Increases good cholesterol. The good cholesterol improves blood flow and the condition of your heart. Ketogenesis helps in the production of the good cholesterol and thus helps in improving heart health.

Improves brain health. Ketone bodies are especially effective as a source of energy for the brain. Many people who have practiced the ketone diet say that it improves their mental clarity and focus.

The Importance of a Well-Balanced Diet

When we talk about a balanced diet, we refer to a variety of foods that supply us with important nutrients such as protein, carbohydrates, healthy fats, vitamins, and minerals. So, what is the importance of a well-balanced diet?

Strengthens immune system. When you consume a diet that's rich in nutrients, your immune system will become stronger. This places your body in a far better place to fight disease vectors that might have otherwise overwhelmed your body's defense system.

Weight loss. In the past, obesity was a problem in only developed nations. Not anymore. Nowadays even poor people are struggling with obesity. This is partially due to fast foods being cheaper and more convenient. As you can imagine, obesity has become a crisis the world over. The open secret is that obesity can be mitigated through a balanced diet. A diet rich in nutritious elements will nourish your body and also regulate your appetite so that you don't fall into the temptation of eating unhealthy foods.

Mental health. People who observe a balanced diet are less likely to fall into bad moods and depression. The nutritious elements stabilize their emotions and enable them to be more resistant to the autosuggestions of their mind.

Skin health. Dry skin is often the result of a bad diet. When you have a balanced diet, your skin and hair are nourished, and it gives you a glow. Foods rich in vitamins and collagen improve skin elasticity.

Promotes growth. A balanced diet helps kids have a well-formed body as they transition into adults and it helps adults maintain a well-figured body.

Summary

A good nutrition is a diet that contains all the important nutrients in appropriate portions. You risk developing complications if you fail to follow a good nutrition. The risk of developing health complications is greatly minimized by a great nutrition. Protein is one of the most important elements of a good nutrition. It is important for muscle health, skin health and development of hair. Protein also plays a role in bodily reactions. Carbohydrates are the major source of energy. They provide glucose that the body cells use to power activities of the body. Fats also play an important role in improving health. Monounsaturated fats and polyunsaturated fats are especially healthy. Vitamins are necessary for the body to function optimally. Minerals and water are important too. People ensure that they have good nutrition to improve their health. They achieve this by consuming foods that are rich in nutritious elements. A high-fat diet promotes strong immunity, better eyesight, a lower risk of heart disease, and stronger bones.

Chapter 15: Exercise

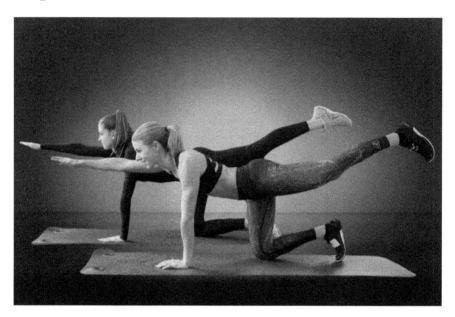

Pros of Exercising While Fasting

For the longest time, it was considered unhealthy to exercise while on a fast, but new evidence has shown that it is perfectly healthy to exercise even while you are fasting.

When you fast for health purposes, it shows that you are committed to improving your health and managing your weight. One of the ways you could get better results is by turning to physical exercise. A combination of intermittent fasting and physical exercise will burn up calories and help you reach your health goals in the shortest time possible.

The time of day that you exercise seems to affect the outcome. For instance, exercising in the morning right after you wake up promotes more weight loss than exercising at night. For intermittent fasting to be effective, you need to abstain from food for at least 16 hours.

When you exercise while on a fast, you speed up weight loss and optimize your health because of increased oxidation that promotes the growth of muscle cells.

It enriches your blood. Exercising has a positive effect on your breathing system and lung capacity. This helps in increasing the oxygen levels in your blood.

Exercising also improves heart health. Aerobic exercises, in particular, improve blood circulation and develop the stamina of the heart. Now, the blood pressure stabilizes and nutrients can spread to the whole body.

Exercising while on a fast improves your body's adaptability. It is never a good idea to idle around while on a fast, as it will trigger cravings. However, when you engage in physical activity, your body starts to adapt. It helps you create more stamina to endure your fast.

Best Exercises to Do

Exercising while fasting increases the rate of calorie burning. As a result, more weight is lost, and health is optimized in much less time. Here are the best exercises to perform while on a fast:

- **Aerobic exercise**

Aerobic exercise increases your heartbeat and breathing cycle. Aerobic exercise also improves lung capacity and heart health. Some of the benefits of aerobic exercise include improved mental health, minimized inflammation, lowered blood pressure, lowered blood sugar, and a minimized risk of heart disease, stroke, type 2 diabetes, and cancer. Aerobic exercises tend to be intense and easy to perform. Some examples of aerobic exercises include dancing, speed-walking, jogging, and cycling.

- **Strength training**

Strength training is important for muscle gain. People who perform strength training have more energy and keep their bodies at peak performance. Strength training improves your mental health, decreases blood sugar levels, enhances weight management, corrects posture, increases balance, and relieves pain in the back and joints. Strength training may be performed either in the gym or at home. Professional guidance depends on the exact exercise and equipment required. Strength training mostly takes the form of exercises such as pull-ups, push-ups, sit-ups, squats, and lunges. It is recommended to take breaks from strength training to allow muscle growth.

- **Stretching**

Stretching exercises are vital in improving the flexibility of a person. The exercises are designed to improve the strength and flexibility of tendons. Stretching exercises also improve the aesthetic quality of muscles. They also improve the circulation of blood and promote nourishment of all body cells.

- **Balance exercises**

Balance exercises promote agility. The exercises are designed to make your joints flexible. Balance exercises lead to improved focus and motor skills. The exercises include squats, sit-ups, and leg lifts.

Summary

Contrary to what people thought for the longest time, it is healthy to exercise while on a fast. A combination of exercise and fasting is a resource-intensive activity that makes your body burn more calories. Studies show that exercising in the morning has a far better outcome than exercising at night before bed. When you exercise while fasting, oxidation in cells promotes the growth of muscles. Exercising while on a fast also enriches your blood. The improved breathing cycle and lung capacity help in increasing the level of oxygen in the blood. Exercising is vital in improving heart health and blood circulation. It is never a good idea to stay idle while you are on a fast. Your hunger will be magnified, and it might cause to break the fast. Some of the best exercises to do for maximum weight loss and health improvement include aerobic exercises, strength training, stretching and balance exercises.

Chapter 16: Having a Partner to Keep You in Check

Role of a Partner

Depriving yourself of food is by no means easy. If you have no experience, the temptation to slide back is real. In some instances, fasting might make you lapse into a worse state than before. This is especially after a small duration of fasting where the hunger is extreme, and then you are tempted into eating unhealthy foods, trapping you into eating them.

Having a partner to keep you in check is a good step, and if they are into fasting themselves, that's even better. Ideally, your partner should be someone that "understands" you. He or she will make fasting less taxing. They will be there to see your progress and offer constructive criticism when needed. As your fasting progresses, they will help you adjust accordingly or make tweaks, to go through the fast in the safest manner possible.

Your partner will hold you accountable for your fasting journey. Attaining health goals is no easy task. It takes dedication, discipline, and consistency. It's exactly why you need a partner to hold you accountable when you stray or when you fall back on your goals. A responsible partner will be interested in your gains (i.e., asking questions about your weight loss so far and wanting to know what your diet is like).

A partner is also important because you have someone to talk to about your journey. They can offer you psychosocial support in your moments of vulnerability. It makes a world of difference. And you will stick to your goals knowing that someone cares.

Traits to Look for in a Partner

Not everyone may qualify to be a partner to someone who's fasting. The first thing to look out for is their opinion on the subject of fasting. Some people seem to think that fasting is a bad practice and a waste of time. Clearly, you wouldn't want such a person as your partner.

- **Patience**

Your partner should demonstrate patience. You cannot rush things while fasting. Sometimes, the results might take time, and in such situations, the last thing you want is someone on your neck, probably trashing your methods.

- **Observation skills**

A great partner must be a good observer. Their job is to spot loopholes that need to be closed, to assess situations, and to weigh overall progress. They need strong observation skills that will make them suitable for their positions. Also, remember that it is sometimes critical to call off a fast. Maybe you will be hard on yourself even when you are falling apart. An observant partner should notice the change and suggest that you stop.

- **Communication skills**

They should have good communication skills. What good is it to know something and not express it in a timely and appropriate fashion? A great partner should be very communicative and should express him/herself in an elaborate manner.

- **Knowledgeable**

A good partner should be knowledgeable. They should have a working knowledge of the whole subject of fasting. During every step of the fast, they should have a mental picture of what's coming. This will strengthen your bond and together you can meet any challenge.

- **Respect**

They should be able to respect you, your methods, and also have self-respect. This creates an enabling environment.

Should You Join A Support Group?

When your brain floods you with hunger hormones during a fast, the temptation to quit is real. One of the methods to minimize your chances of quitting is to join a support group. This is ideally a group of people who have similar fasting pursuits as you. Now you have a family to keep you in check and boost your confidence.

A support network will allow you to cope and express your feelings and get connected with like-minded people. In times of vulnerability, others will come to your help. As other members share their experiences, you learn that you are not alone, and you even broaden your perspective and wisdom.

Support networks include people who are at various stages toward the common goal you all have. In times of conflict, you have ready help, and if you are at an advanced stage yourself, then you should offer help to those in need of it too. Support networks have non-judgmental environments and therapeutic effects.

The best support groups are those that foster frequent get-togethers. Ideally, the members should come from the same society, but that doesn't mean other kinds of support groups are necessary. For instance, you could join an online support network and be free to commune with your family at your convenience. Online support groups seem to be a thing nowadays. People from around the world with common goals are coming together to form support networks.

The most important thing when you join a support group is to become a giver rather than a taker. Or both. When everyone is interested in giving, you have a resourceful group of like-minded people.

Summary

People who are overwhelmed by the idea of staying without food should consider getting a partner. Your partner should help you cultivate a strong sense of discipline and stick to your routine. Ideally, your partner should be someone who understands you. He or she will help you get through fasting. A supportive partner is there to check your progress and offer constructive criticism when the occasion calls for it. He or she should be someone that you can open up to and express your fears and concerns. With the right partner, your fasting journey will be smooth and enjoyable. Your partner should be patient, observant, communicative, respectful, and knowledgeable. Joining a support group will help you come together with other like-minded people for a common goal. You are guaranteed of ready help and psychosocial support. The best support group to join should comprise of people from your local area, but it doesn't rule out joining even online support groups and communing with people from different parts of the world.

Chapter 17: Motivation

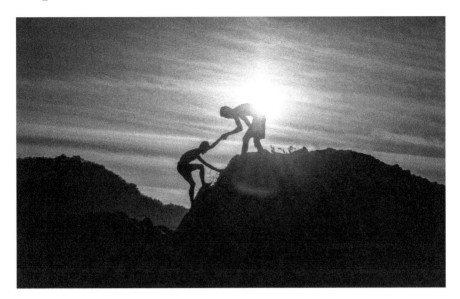

How to Stay Motivated Throughout Your Fast

Get a partner. If you go it alone, you are much more likely to forgive yourself and tweak the fast to suit you. For that reason, let there be a person to whom you are accountable. This person should put you in check and ensure that you follow the rules. Offer constructive criticism, and suggestions. A partner will help you stick to your routine. The ideal partner should be patient, empathetic, a good communicator, and knowledgeable about fasting. Let them share in your accomplishments as much as they have shared in your trials and struggle.

Seek knowledge. Being informed makes all the difference. You will know every possible outcome. You are aware of all the side effects of fasting and how to persist through the unpleasant experience instead of just quitting. Knowledge will help you optimize your fast and make you reap more benefits than anyone who had just deprived themselves of food. Being knowledgeable is important also in the sense that you are more aware of when to stop.

Set goals. Don't get into fasting with mental blindness. Instead, make an effort to set milestones. When you achieve a goal—for instance, when you hit your target weight—celebrate and then go back to reducing weight. Your brain responds to victory by making you feel confident. Now, you will have more confidence in your capacity to withstand hunger.

Develop positivity. A positive attitude makes all the difference. Keep reading about successful people who have achieved what you are looking for. Lockout all the negative energies that would derail you.

Record your progress. It is easy to underestimate yourself. As long as you keep going, the achievements will always be there. It's just a matter of recognizing them and celebrating.

How to Make Fasting Your Lifestyle

There are different approaches to fasting. You may fast every other day, once a week, or even a couple of times every month. In each instance, there are benefits.

But if you'd like to reap great benefits out of fasting, you should purposefully make it a daily ritual. Many people in the world today fast on a daily basis and have reported an increased quality of life.

The most common and most rewarding method is the 16:8 intermittent fasting. In this method, you fast for 16 hours in a day and then eat during the other 8 hours to complete the cycle.

Ideally, when you wake up, you should take a drink of water or black coffee and either exercise or just go on about your work. At around noon, your eating window opens, and you're free to have your meals up until 8 pm when the eating window closes.

During this eight-hour eating window, it is common to be tempted to overeat or indulge in unhealthy foods, thinking that the coming fast will "take care of that." Well, you must be careful not to fall into this temptation, or else your gains will be negated. Consume healthy and nutritious foods during the eating window and adhere to your 16-hour fast. The weight loss starts occurring in as short a span as a few days.

If you incorporate intermittent fasting into your lifestyle, the weight loss keeps going until you hit a stable weight where it plateaus. When fasting is your lifestyle, it makes your health improvement and weight loss permanent.

Summary

You need to take a few measures to stay motivated throughout the fast. One of the measures is to get a partner. A partner should hold you accountable and keep you in check so that you don't stray from the fasting routine. The ideal partner should be patient, empathetic, and a good communicator. Another way of motivating yourself is through seeking knowledge. As a knowledgeable person, you will be aware of all the responses that your body will give off. Knowledge will also help you optimize your fast and get the best possible results. Other ways to stay motivated throughout the fast include setting goals, developing positivity and recording your progress. If you make fasting part of your lifestyle, you stand to reap more benefits. The most common and most efficient fasting method is the 16:8, where you fast for 16 hours and then have an eating window of 8 hours.

Chapter 18: Foods for the Fast

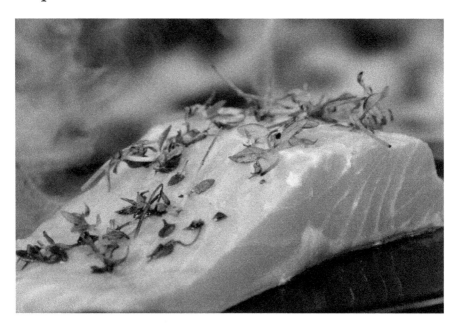

How Food Controls the Rate of the Success of Fasting

Depriving yourself of food is no easy task. Your body will tune up the hunger, and you will have to suppress the urge to feed. Not easy.

When you consume food, it is digested and released into the bloodstream as sugars. The pancreas secretes the hormone insulin to help in absorption of these sugars into body cells. When you stay for long without eating, there is no more food getting digested, and thus no more sugars getting released into the blood. The body soon runs out of the existing sugars and meets a crisis. The body is forced to switch to fats to provide energy for various physiological functions.

The foods that you eat have a massive impact on the efficacy of the fast. If you take light meals or small portions of food during the eating window, you will experience a higher degree of hunger during the fast. On the other side, if you consume large amounts of food during your eating window, your hunger will not be as intense.

One of the tricks to reducing hunger during the fast is to consume foods that are high in dietary fiber. Such foods make you full for a long time and will thus minimize the unpleasant feeling triggered by hunger.

Consuming healthy foods during your eating window is important. Some people fall into the temptation of eating unhealthy foods or even eating too much, and the effect is negative.

Intermittent fasting is favored by many people because it doesn't restrict consumption of foods, unlike fad diets that insist on vegan meals or raw food.

The Worst Foods to Take During Fasting

If you want to speed up your weight loss and avoid lifestyle diseases, these are some of the foods to cut back on, or maybe stay away from:

Sugary drinks. The high dose of fructose in sugary drinks will cause an extreme surge of blood sugar levels. High amounts of this kind of sugar promote insulin resistance and liver disease. High levels of insulin resistance have a negative impact on the absorption of sugars into body cells. This creates the perfect recipe for the development of heart disease and diabetes.

Junk food. They might taste heavenly, but the ingredients of most junk foods come from hell. Junk foods have almost zero nutritional value. Fries are prepared using hydrogenated oil that contains trans fats. Studies have been made on trans fats, and the conclusion is that continued consumption of trans fats leads to heart complications and cancer.

Processed food. Most processed foods have a long shelf life thanks to a host of nasty chemicals poured into them. The processed foods are made durable to gain a commercial edge over organic products with a limited shelf life. Most processed foods are high in sugars, sodium, and have low fiber content and nutrients.

White bread and cakes. Baked goods tend to affect people with celiac disease, most especially. But more than that, most of these baked goods are stashed with processed ingredients—sugars and fats—and they are low on fiber. Most baked goods trigger abnormal surges in blood sugar levels and increase the risk of heart disease.

Alcohol. Studies show that alcohol induces inflammation on the liver. Excessive alcohol consumption will eliminate all the successes of your fast and promote weight gain and even development of diabetes.

Seed oils. Studies show that these oils are unnatural. They contain harmful fatty acids that increase the risk of developing heart complications.

The Best Foods to Take During Fasting

These are some of the best foods to indulge in while you fast to reach your important health goals:

Nuts. Nuts are rich in nutritional value. Almonds, Brazil nuts, lentils, oatmeal, etc. have properties that help in the production of good cholesterol. Good cholesterol promotes heart health. Nuts are excellent sources of vitamins and minerals. Oatmeal, in particular, is essential in normalizing blood glucose levels.

Fruits and greens. They are important sources of essential nutrients that improve both gut health and brain health. Broccoli is rich in phytonutrients that reduce the risk of heart complications and cancers. Apples contain antioxidants that eliminate harmful radicals. Kale contains the vital vitamin K. Blueberries are excellent sources of fiber and phytonutrients. Avocados are good sources of monounsaturated fats that lower bad cholesterol and improve heart health.

White meats. These are an excellent source of protein and fatty acids. Fish provide omega-3 fatty acids which improve heart health and stimulate muscle growth. Chicken is a great source of protein, and it promotes the growth of muscle cells.

Grains. They are excellent sources of protein and dietary fiber that will keep you full. Grains also help in improving heart health and normalizing blood pressure.

Eggs. Eggs are excellent sources of protein, and they tend to fill you up thus minimizing hunger levels.

Tubers. Foods such as potatoes and sweet potatoes are loaded with essential vitamins and carbohydrates.

Dairy. Dairy seems to reduce the risk of development of obesity and type 2 diabetes. Cheese and whole milk are excellent sources of protein and essential minerals that promote bone development.

Summary

When you go on a fast, your body increases the hunger levels in an attempt to pressure you to look for food. Staying without food for a long time causes the body to switch to fats as an alternative energy source. When the carbohydrates supplying energy to the brain are depleted, the liver produces ketone bodies to supply energy to the brain. The food you eat (and the portion) will impact your hunger levels during the fast. It is important to consume healthy foods during the eating window no matter how strong the temptation to stray is. Some of the worst foods that you can indulge in while fasting includes sugary drinks, junk foods, processed foods, white bread and cakes, alcohol, and seed oils. On the other hand, some of the best foods you can indulge in would be nuts, fruits and greens, white meat, grains, eggs, tubes, and dairy.

PART 3

Chapter 1: What Is the Ketogenic Diet

In this first chapter, we are going to discuss what the ketogenic diet is and why it is becoming more and more popular these days. In fact, you can browse the web for a few minutes, and you will easily find articles and blogs dedicated to this topic. Most people, however, decide to follow the diet without actually knowing what they are getting themselves into and are not able to distinguish good information from harmful ones. This is why we decided to start off the book by laying out the foundation of this diet, so everybody will understand its principles. Let us get started!

If there is a diet that is often misunderstood it is the ketogenic diet. Publicized by some as a very effective means of weight loss, criticized by others for the supposed — and often exaggerated — risks associated with it. It is actually an important tool, especially when it comes to improving one's health. Any particular diet that must be used with due precautions, but the keto diet can guarantee effective results where other methods often fail.

The idea on which the ketogenic diet is based is the ability of our body to use lipid reserves with great effectiveness when the availability of carbohydrates is greatly reduced. The physiological mechanisms activated in this situation reduce the possible use of proteins for energy, protecting the lean mass and significantly reducing the sensation of hunger.

In the clinical field, the first documented use of a ketogenic diet to treat specific diseases dates back to the 1920s when Russell Wilder used it to control attacks in pediatric patients with epilepsy that could not be treated with drugs. The keto diet became the center of attention again in the 1990s, and since then, the usage of the diet increased. In the 60s and 70s, with the constant increase of obesity among the populace, numerous studies were carried out on the use of a low-calorie diet that could lead to rapid and significant weight reduction without affecting the lean mass.

The various protocols of PSMF (Protein Sparing Modified Fast) were born, these are diets characterized by a reduced protein intake with a near-total absence of carbohydrates and a measured protein intake aimed at minimizing the loss of precious muscle mass. The implementation of the ketogenic diet saw a surge with the appearance of low-carb diets and do-it-yourself diets on the market, such as the Atkins diet. Although, that is a shameful model that drastically reduces the consumption of carbohydrates instead so one can freely eat fat and proteins. The Atkins diet is a grotesque caricature of the ketogenic diet based on improbable and fanciful interpretations of human physiology, which is why it was rightly criticized by the entire scientific community.

Recently, the emergence of the Paleo diet has brought attention back to food regimens that emphasize reduced carbohydrate content to generate ketosis. Here, solid scientific basis intertwines with perturbed, poorly-engineered biological concepts that have often generated ineffective solutions where every carbohydrate is disregarded and considered a poison, while the consumption of bacon is recommended, as it was the staple diet during the Paleolithic era. Now, there has been a renewed interest within the scientific community towards this diet, starting with the investigation on the use of the ketogenic diet for the treatment of obesity and other medical conditions or issues such as the formation of tumors, neurological diseases like Alzheimer's and Parkinson's disease, diabetes, and metabolic syndrome as well.

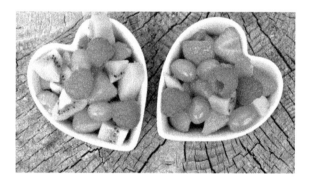

The human body has several ways to accumulate energy reserves, the most consistent of which is through the use of adipose tissue (fat). An average individual weighing 70 kg, can have as much as 15 kg of adipose tissue, while the carbohydrate portion amounts to little less than half a kilogram. It is evident that sugar reserves can guarantee energy for very limited periods of time, while fats represent a huge reserve of energy. Tissues receive energy in proportion to the actual availability of substrates in the blood. When glucose is present in sufficient quantities, it appears to be the most preferred energy source used by all of the body's tissues. When glucose is in short supply, most organs and tissues can use fatty acids as an energy source, or they convert other substances into sugars, especially some amino acids like alanine and glutamine, through a process called gluconeogenesis.

Some organs and tissues like the brain, central nervous system, red blood cells, and type II muscle fibers cannot use free fatty acids. But, when the body experiences glucose deficiency, they can use ketone bodies. These are substances derived from lipidic parts, the concentration of which is usually very small under normal conditions but increase considerably in particular situations, such as a prolonged fasting or a long period without carbohydrate consumption.

The increase in the concentration of ketone bodies in the blood, resulting from fasting or severe reduction of their food intake with the diet, is a completely natural condition called ketosis. This is a mechanism that was developed to help us cope with the stringent metabolic needs and limited availability of food back when our ancestors lived in a hunter-gatherer society. This process also naturally occurs in the morning after fasting overnight or after an intense and vigorous physical activity.

The severe restriction of carbohydrate intake through the action of hormones such as insulin and glucagon promotes the mobilization of lipids from the reserve tissues and their use as fuel. Given the scarcity of glucose, the present Acetyl-CoA is used for the production of ketone bodies while substances such as acetone, acetoacetate, and β-hydroxybutyric acid, become the preferred fuel for the cells of the central nervous system. During ketosis, blood sugar is maintained at normal levels thanks to the presence of glucogenic amino acids and, above all, glycerol, which is derived from the demolition of triglycerides for the formation of glucose.

In physiological ketosis, the presence of ketone bodies in the blood passes from 0.1 mmol/dl to about 7 mmol/dl. The significant alteration of the body's pH levels, which normally stays around 7.4 but could decrease slightly in the first few days given the acidity of ketone bodies, may return quickly to normal levels as long as the concentration of ketone bodies remains below 10 mmol/dl.

The effect of saving protein reserves could occur through different mechanisms which is why the use of proteins is important during the first few days of the diet. But, as the body begins to predominantly use free fatty acids and ketones for their energy needs, the demand for glucose drops drastically, accompanied by the reduction of the use of amino acids for energy purposes. A direct effect of the ketone bodies on protein metabolism and on the functions of the thyroid is not excluded, a noticeable effect is the reduction of T3.

The excess ketones are eliminated through breathing in the form of acetone, which induces what we refer to as 'acetone breath,' and through the urine, where excess acidity is buffered by simultaneous elimination of sodium, potassium, and magnesium.

Ketosis introduces changes in the concentration of different hormones and nutrients, including ghrelin, amylin, leptin and, of course, ketone bodies themselves. It is probably through these variations that one of the most relevant effects of the ketogenic diet is initiated: the reduction or total disappearance of the sensation of hunger. This is undoubtedly a situation that better helps one to endure the typical rigor of this diet.

Chapter 2: The Three Principles of the Ketogenic Diet

The ketogenic diet is based on 3 essential concepts:

Reduction of simple and complex carbohydrates

Foods containing carbohydrates must be totally eliminated, even if this is practically impossible. The portions of the vegetables which contain fructose are maintained, resulting in the collapse of complex carbohydrates in favor of the simple ones which are very low in quantity. These nutrients are used as a primary energy source by most organisms. When they're reduced to a minimum, the body is then forced to dispose of excess fat reserves. Moreover, carbohydrates are nutrients that significantly stimulate insulin (anabolic and fattening hormones), so their moderation should also have metabolic significance.

Partial increase of fats and a percentage of proteins to keep the increase of calories constant

After eliminating the carbohydrates, consumption of protein-rich foods should be kept constant, as well as foods with a high content of fats (oils, oil seeds, oily fleshy fruits, etc.). In theory, this compensates for the caloric reduction of glucose thanks to the greater quantity of lipids. In practice, for obvious reasons like appetite (or hunger), it is necessary to increase the portions and frequency of the consumption of protein sources.

Some justify this 'correction' by stating that more proteins are useful for conserving lean mass. It should be specified, however, that many amino acids are glucogenic (they are converted into glucose by neoglucogenesis) and have a metabolic action similar to carbohydrates, partially negating the effect on lipolytic enzymes and lessening the production of ketone bodies (see below). Moreover, in clinical practice, the menu of the ketogenic diet is never normocaloric and provides less energy than necessary. Which is why, before you venture into such a strict regimen, you should try a well-balanced calorie diet first.

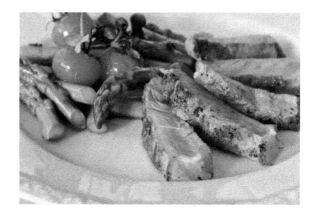

Production of ketone bodies

The hepatic neoglucogenesis necessary to synthesize glucose (starting from certain amino acids and glycerol) is not fast enough to cover the daily glucose needs of the body. At the same time, fat oxidation (closely related to and dependent on glycolysis) 'jams' and causes the accumulation of intermediate molecules called ketone bodies. These ketones, which at physiological concentrations are easily disposable, in the ketogenic diet reach levels that are toxic for the tissues.

Toxic does not necessarily mean poisonous, but rather, it is something which causes intoxication. This effect is clearly distinguishable by the reduction of appetite, that is, the anorectic effect on the brain. Although, like the heart, the nervous tissue can partially use the ketone bodies to generate energy.

A healthy organism can function with high quantities of ketone bodies in the blood since the excess is eliminated (we do not know how much effort is required by the body to accomplish this) through renal filtration. Obviously, people suffering from certain pathologies (defects in insulin secretion that's typical of type 1 diabetes, renal failure which is also triggered by advanced type 2 diabetes, liver failure, etc.) have a very high risk of developing metabolic acidosis or diabetic ketoacidosis, risking coma or even death.

Chapter 3: An Example of the Ketogenic Diet Meal Plan

Now it is time to dive right into the core of the ketogenic diet. Here are some of the meals that you can try to start off with:

Breakfast

- A protein source:

  o Eggs

  o 50 g of meat preserved as bacon, raw ham, or bresaola

- 25 - 50 g of carbohydrates

  o Rye bread

  o Dried fruit

  o Pistachios

  o Peanuts

  o Peanut butter

- 30g of fat

  o Low-carbohydrate and high-fat cheese

  o Flakes

  o Milk

  o Butter

Mid-morning snack

A mid-morning snack can provide a modest intake of carbohydrates that can be taken from these choices

- Two teaspoons of peanut butter and celery

- 50g of dried fruit

- Toasted pistachios

- Almonds

- Toasted peanuts

Lunch

During the week, lunch can take the form of the any of the following:

- A protein source of about 200 - 250 g:

    o Fish like salmon or trout or tuna

    o Meat like chicken or turkey

- A portion of 100 - 200 g of vegetables:

    o Salad

    o Green beans

    o Salad rocket

    o Lettuce

    o Asparagus

- o Mushrooms

- o Broccoli

- o Peas

- A source of fat of about 25g:

  - o Olive oil

  - o Butter

  - o Mayonnaise

  - o Cream

Mid-afternoon snack

Alternate the following foods during the week:

- A source of fat, around 50 - 100 g:

  - o Cheese

  - o Flakes

  - o Milk

- A protein source or a modest source of carbohydrates:

  - o Vegetable soup

  - o Carrots

  - o Peas

Dinner

During the week, dinner can be eaten through any of the following:

- A protein source of about 150 - 200 g:
    - Meat such as hamburger, veal, or goat
    - Fish such as trout, salmon, tuna, or swordfish
    - Eggs
- A source of fat of around 20 - 30 g:
    - Cheese
    - Oil
    - Butter
    - Bacon
- A portion of vegetables of about 200 g:
    - Salad
    - String beans
    - Rocket salad
    - Lettuce
    - Asparagus
    - Mushrooms
    - Broccoli
    - Tomatoes
    - Peppers
    - Peas

Chapter 4: Two Types of Ketogenic Diet

There are two main types of ketogenic diet: the intermittent ketogenic diet and the cyclic ketogenic diet. There is also a whole series of diets that follow the same basic principle of the ketogenic diet, which is weight loss obtained through the action of the ketogenic bodies. In this final chapter, we will take a look at the two main types of ketogenic diet.

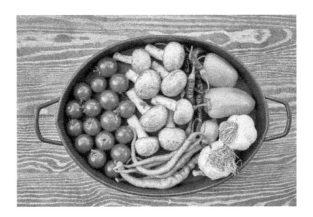

Cyclic ketogenic diet

It is the most widely used type of ketogenic diet, and it is divided into two different phases. The first phase lasts about 5 - 6 days and includes a low-carbohydrate intake in the diet, as well as a recharging phase that has a duration of 1 - 2 days, which requires carbohydrate consumption to be very high. In this way, the muscle glycogen reserves are replenished for a whole week during the refill phase. In the second phase, 10 - 12 grams of carbohydrates per kg of body weight must be consumed each and every day.

Intermittent ketogenic diet

This ketogenic diet is a type of diet followed a lot by athletes in general, but not by those who practice sports like bodybuilding, in which the activity is aimed at increasing muscle mass. In this diet, the body supplies muscle glycogen stores, which makes it suitable for those who practice aerobic exercises. The carbohydrate refilling phase takes place during the entire week, and each meal is recommended to provide at least 0.7 g of carbohydrates for every kilogram of body weight.

CPSIA information can be obtained
at www.ICGtesting.com
Printed in the USA
LVHW081754061120
670969LV00012B/1540